THREE-TIME
AWARD WINNER!

2023 Florida Authors and Publishers Association

WINNER!
How to/Self-Help

2023 Florida Authors and Publishers Association

WINNER!
Health

2023 Florida Authors and Publishers Association

WINNER!
Fitness/Sports/Recreation

Aqua Therapy How I prevented Major Surgery and Got My Life Back

Published in the United States by
JMC INVESTMENT PARTNERS, LLC

First published April 2023
ISBN: 979-8-9882820-0-6

Health, Fitness, and surgery prevention.

Website: www.howIpreventedmajorsurgery.com

Email: john@howipreventedmajorsurgery.com

What People are Saying about this Book!

"I have lived with chronic pain in my lower back for over 15 years. I have resisted the urge to have surgery but have tried everything from physical therapy to chiropractic to cortisone injections. There has been no long-lasting pain relief.... until now.

"When I began using the aqua exercises detailed in John's new book; the almost-immediate results have been nothing short of amazing. My back pain has diminished almost completely.

"However, it does come back if I work in the yard, but each time I
do my therapy, it gets better, and my back and core are feeling much stronger. I am also currently not taking any pain meds. I strongly recommend this program."

—*Randy Miller, Media Professional and Host, The National Defense Military Radio Show.*

"I have personally witnessed the success that John Capozzi has achieved through his dedication to the aqua therapy program he created. It's been my honor to assist him in the creation of the exercises he is sharing with others who are seeking to decrease their pain and improve their well-being."
—Jea Coffman, ACE Certified Personal Trainer, AFAA Certified Group Exercise Instructor, 500 hours of Experienced Yoga Teaching, registered with the Yoga Alliance. www.thaiyogafit.com Teaching, registered with the Yoga Alliance. www.thaiyogafit.com

"Aqua Therapy has many benefits without the negative effects that land-based training has when it comes to both training and for preventing injuries. By unloading the joints and allowing gentle progressive strengthening in omnidirectional patterns, we give our fascial system the opportunity to create structural tensegrity which is paramount for long term injury resiliency and preventative care and maintenance of our body throughout life.

It's through a structured program like this that we can prevent these kinds of major surgeries and alter the course of someone's life.

—Austin Jensen, CSCA, PTA, LMT, former Division I football player

"Mr. Capozzi has been a patient of the Lerner Cohen medical practice for many years. Over the years his back condition became worse and the surgical specialists he met with strongly suggested advanced surgery to fuse his back. Normally I would consider surgery for a patient if I felt it was totally needed.

However, in Mr. Capozzi's case, his back condition was severely advanced, and his surgery would require at least 8 hours of anesthesia with months of recovery. I was deeply concerned that at his age, his risks were enormous. But when he told me that he had investigated aqua therapy and wanted to try strengthening his core to see if it might help him at least function again, I was very pleased.

He certainly had nothing to lose. I am elated to know that his program has worked.

Given his success, I am using his program myself, as I too have a bad back, but I have also recommended it to several of my older patients. I believe that if a patient can avoid major surgery, that's a very good thing."

—Dr. Brad Lerner, Principal, Lerner Cohen, Sarasota, FL. www.lernercohen.com

"Aqua therapy How I prevented Major Surgery" has been a godsend to both my wife and I in terms of helping us strengthen our core and alleviate back pain. Highly effective!"
James Stavridis, PhD; Admiral, US Navy (Retired); Former Supreme Allied Commander of NATO; Chairman of the Board of Trustees, the Rockefeller Foundation.

"For many years I have been a licensed home care representative and a trained health practitioner for patients with Dementia and Alzheimer. I am currently using John Capozzi's Aqua Therapy book for my patients to prevent atrophy and to maintain strength.

The results with all my patients have been exceptional. However, with my dementia patients the results have been nothing short of incredible.

Not only are these patients happier in the pool, but they look forward to our session's days in advance.

Most importantly, I am seeing actual results. They are feeling better physically.

Tamara Andelkovic. Licensed home care service representative; Home Instead Senior Care Company.

Foreword
By Dr. Bruce Becker

This book is a single individual's story about his experiences with severe spine pain and his ultimate salvation using aquatic therapy. In my discussions with John, I relayed that while his personal story, while striking, is far from unique. The uses of aquatic immersion for healing dates to prehistory, forming the basis of many ancient communities around springs and other water sources. Ancient Romans extensively built and used their elaborate baths for healing, social gathering, and hygiene.

Spas were used in early America for all these same reasons.

American medicine made significant use of medical hydrology for the treatment of many diseases during the 1800s through mid-20th century but for a number of reasons, medical science has largely ignored this history. Physical therapists no longer have aquatic therapy training as a mandated curriculum component, nor is exposure to aquatic therapy part of medical school or residency training.

In my clinical practice of Physical Medicine and Rehabilitation, I have referred many hundreds of my patients for aquatic therapy. I have had opportunity to work with many Olympic-level elite athletes and recommended aquatic cross-training as a component of their competitive training to reduce joint injuries, build balance and strength, and increase cardio-respiratory function. (1) I've researched aquatic therapy from a medical standpoint, written and published on it, and lectured globally. I'm a devout believer in the unique value of aquatic exercise and immersion for healing and health promotion.

The response of the human body to the aquatic environment is profound. Perhaps it is because all of us spent the initial formative months of our lives immersed in a warm-water pool of amniotic fluid that we can so readily sink into a pool with relief. Mother Nature knew that this was the environment that would provide protection and the optimum conditions for growth during this critical period.

But the combined effects of all the properties of water, from buoyancy, through hydrostatic pressure, to its thermal conductive properties make the aquatic environment tremendously useful and effective for health recovery, for health maintenance and for recreation.

The physiologic benefits of aquatic exercise and immersion are truly profound. (2) Aquatic immersion has been shown scientifically to positively affect cardiac function and improve circulation, while also producing forces that can aid in increasing respiratory strength and endurance. Aquatic immersion improves circulation and muscle blood flow, aiding in oxygen delivery to injured and healing tissues. Even the Greeks and Romans understood that it improves kidney function, aiding in elimination of metabolic waste products.

Recent research has shown that immersion in water produces a positive effect upon the central nervous system that might aid in the management of depression, post-traumatic stress disorder (PTSD,) and maybe even in learning disorders. It has been shown to improve brain function in dementia and many neurologic diseases like Parkinsonism. (3)

Recent research has shown that immersion in water produces a positive effect upon the central nervous system that might aid in the management of depression, post-traumatic stress disorder (PTSD,) and maybe even in learning disorders. It has been shown to improve brain function in dementia and many neurologic diseases like Parkinsonism. (3)

John's story began with his severe spine pain pathology. Because aquatic immersion produces an effective offloading of body weight due to buoyancy. Water is denser than the human body, and therefore at waist level immersion depth, the hips, knees ankles and feet have about a 50% reduction in loading due to buoyancy and at mid-chest depth, about 75% offloading.

At neck depth, as in deep water exercise and immersion, there is essentially no gravity - loading of the lumbar spine and only the weight of the head on the cervical spine. As a result, this effect may be used to excellent clinical benefit in facilitating recovery from training or rehabilitating from a lower extremity or spine injury. I have seen the impact of this immediate offloading on my patients with severe spine pain many times, and on several occasions, even found them in tears because their pain was so dramatically reduced.

Years ago, a former NFL All-Pro linebacker was referred to me for rehab. He was a massive human being, 6' 8" tall, weighing nearly 300 pounds, almost none of which was fat. He had sustained a severe lumbar spine injury while working for USAID in Nairobi, and on evaluation was found to have severe spinal stenosis, multiple levels of disc loss, and nerve compressions of several spinal nerves.

He had seen several neurosurgeons, all recommending multiple level surgical decompression, spinal fusions, and instrumentation, all of which might mean still scant improvement and considerable risk of persistent pain. I watched his initial response to immersion in a deep-water therapy pool. He teared up, stating his back pain was almost completely gone.

We began an aggressive aquatic therapy program progressing him from just floating, to deep water walking, then running, doing cross-country skiing movements, and including core strengthening exercises all in deep water.

After a month, he returned home to his ranch in eastern Oregon, and dug a deep hole with a backhoe for a deep-water exercise pool, using a polyethylene circular septic tank with the end cut off, plumbing it for heating and filtration! He has never needed surgery and still uses the "hot tub septic tank."

I've seen similar results in many patients with spinal stenosis over the years since then, and while I cannot explain the anatomic reasons for these results, the improvement in function and pain reduction has been nearly universal. Many research studies have supported my clinical observations. (4, 5, 6)

The medical value of aquatic therapy has been better understood in recent years, but unfortunately it still does not come first to mind for many physicians.

The physical properties of water, combined with the human physiologic response to immersion make the aquatic environment almost uniquely beneficial in the management of patients with spine dysfunction. It's safe for patient with extremely low levels of fitness, or highly obese patients, both difficult populations to treat on land.

I jokingly (but somewhat seriously) tell my physical therapists that if I had to choose between a pool for my patients and a therapist, I'd choose the pool. Fortunately, this is rarely the dilemma.

John has developed his own regimen of spine exercises through trial and error, but a skilled therapist can be very useful in adapting an effective exercise and rehabilitative regimen to nearly any aquatic environment. Over the past 25 years, there are many physical therapists who have trained in the principles of aquatic therapy, many of them using my textbook *(Comprehensive Aquatic Therapy, 3rd Ed .)*

Most communities have someone with this experience. The pool is a highly forgiving environment, appropriate to folks with spine pain very early in their recovery as well as for long-term spine health maintenance.

REFERENCES

1. Becker BE, Lindle-Chewning JM, Huff K, Sherlock BW, Sherlock LA. Aquatic Cross Training for Athletes: Part 1. *Strength & Conditioning Journal (Lippincott Williams & Wilkins).* 2008; 30(2):18-26.

2. Becker BE. Aquatic Therapy: Scientific Foundations and Clinical Rehabilitation Applications. *PM&R.* 2009; 1(9):859-872.

3. Becker BE. Aquatic Therapy in Contemporary Neurorehabilitation: An Update. *PM R.* Dec 2020;12(12):1251-1259.

4. Dundar U, Solak O, Yigit I, Evcik D, Kavuncu V. Clinical effectiveness of aquatic exercise to treat chronic low back pain: a randomized controlled trial. *Spine (Phila Pa 1976).* Jun 15 2009; 34(14):1436-1440.

5. Simmerman SM, Sizer PS, Dedrick GS, Apte GG, Brismee JM. Immediate changes in spinal height and pain after aquatic vertical traction in patients with persistent low back symptoms: a crossover clinical trial. *PM R.* May 2011; 3(5):447-457.

6. Becker B, Cole A. *Comprehensive Aquatic Therapy, 3rd Ed.* Pullman WA: Washington State University Publishing; 2011.

The Author's Story

By age 77, John Capozzi already had three back surgeries … but he was diagnosed in 2020 with a new and terribly damaged spine condition. Three of the top orthopedic surgeons in America recommended that he have "major" back surgery to repair multiple discs. A herniation. The need for a fusion.   A titanium plate screwed into two vertebrae. And require almost a year of recovery to learn how to walk again. Due to his new back problem, John's quality of life had diminished significantly, and even simple tasks such as putting on his socks and shoes without help became almost impossible. Sleeping flat in a bed was also impossible, so he was forced to sleep in a chair for several months.

However, John was advised by his primary physician that, while in most cases he recommended surgery when the facts warrant it, in

John's case—given his age and the magnitude of the proposed surgery—that John consider alternative solutions to reduce his excruciating pain and his almost total lack of mobility. This advice led to him researching non-surgical treatments.

He tested a variety of exercises and stretches but ruled out many for fear they might further stress or damage his back.

However, each of the exercises contained in this book has been tested by John with a goal of strengthening his core and stretching specific muscles and ligaments, such as his hamstrings, which influence the lower back.

As you will read in this book, John had a long history with martial arts. He also participated in many professional and leisure sports activities. His sports activities, which started in his high school years, are also considered a contributor to his bad back.

In 2020, his back totally lost its ability to function to the extent that John could not sleep in a prone condition; he had to sleep in a chair. He could not walk more than 10 or 20 feet without sitting down to reduce the pain. If he was able to reach his mailbox, he had to sit on the sidewalk for five or 10 minutes to regain enough strength to simply return home.

Since he could no longer walk his dog on a leash, walking his dog represented opening the back door of his home and without a leash, telling the dog to go outside to "do your business." If the dog did not return, then that would be the end of the dog.

The task of "walking the dog" became even more daunting at night because his neighborhood in Florida has a significant coyote and bobcat problem due to the extensive building in the area and the loss of their natural habitat.

His neighborhood had already lost two dogs and a cat to coyotes. As such, "walking the dog" came with carrying a 9mm Glock handgun to the door to provide "cover" for dog, in the event he was attacked.

His options to try to return to some semblances of normalcy were more surgery or to start on opioid drugs to manage the pain. Additionally, it appeared that his condition, even with more surgery, would never allow him to exercise, ride his bike, or work in the yard again. His surgeons counseled him that even with a very successful surgical outcome, he would forever have a significant reduction in his mobility and quality of life. Driving his car for any distance would probably be difficult if not impossible.

The three orthopedic surgeons that John consulted with were three of the top orthopedic surgeons in America. After each reviewed his most current MRIs and X-rays, they all came to the exact same conclusion: he would need a fusion using a titanium plate with multiple titanium screws.

The surgery would require a back incision of about six to eight inches, take about eight hours of anesthesia, and would require two surgeons working together: one to hold the plate in place while the other administered the screws into his spine. His recovery would take six to eight months while wearing a massive brace.

A copy of his medical evaluation is included in Chapter Two. However, given his age, John's primary physician strongly suggested that he consider pain medications sufficient to allow him to partially function and avoid yet another major surgery that would require eight hours of anesthesia and a very lengthy and difficult recovery.

So, three days before his scheduled procedure, John decided to cancel his surgery.

He then embarked upon a research campaign to see if there might be an alternative solution that would allow him to achieve a measure of pain reduction, mobility, and avoid the highly risky surgery.

Another goal was to avoid the use of opioids for pain relief. His research led him to a military physical therapist who served in the Middle East and who cared for disabled veterans.

She advised him to investigate "aqua therapy" to strengthen his core, in the hope that a stronger core might offer a measure of pain relief for his back.

So, John was given a suggestion to explore aqua therapy by a physical therapist. He then spent the next several months investigating "aqua therapy." His research revealed that as people aged, many failed to maintain core strength, and the loss of core strength can contribute to a variety of problems, a weak back being one of them.

Further research concluded that aqua therapy might be valuable in strengthening a person's core, which in turn might offer protection for the spine and help reduce pain. Following this research and after experimentation, he created the exercise program contained in this book.

Once John developed his program, he then religiously used his therapy program every day, rain, or shine, and after several months, he achieved a significant reduction in his back pain. After over a year of daily aqua therapy, he regained an over 95% reduction in pain and a range of motion so incredible that he could walk great distances, ride his bike, work in his yard, and sleep again in his bed.

John believes that being in a pool and being "weightless" with minimal pounding, if any, on the spine would cause almost ZERO risks or downsides from the use of such therapy to attempt to cure his back pain. Of importance to every reader of this book, John knew that if his program did not work for him, as a last resort he could always reconsider surgery.

Question:
So, why did I write this book?

Answer:

When I started my aqua therapy program I had put all the exercises on white pieces of paper that I printed for my personal use. But once several neighbors read the program, they asked for copies.   Then I asked my personal physician to review my program to ensure he was ok with what I wanted to do … and to give me his approval. My physician not only gave his approval, but said he wanted to use my program himself as he also has a bad back.

That caused me to consider writing a book because as I did more research, I found that there are many hundreds of millions of people in the world who are suffering from atrophy. Many are confined to wheelchairs from accidents and illness. Others are grossly overweight and simply can't exercise.   Others have broken bones or were born with physical defects that prevent them from exercising.

But I'm living proof that aqua therapy, aqua yoga, and aqua stretching can be done by "everyone" using a pool. Exercises for just about every part of a body can be performed easily and without serious risk of injury. As you will read, not only did I solve a serious problem without surgery, I learned that aqua therapy could prevent atrophy.

A Doctor's Report

Orthopedic Center
May 15th, 2020
#345123, Capozzi, John

Mr. Capozzi is a very pleasant 78-year-old gentleman who has come to me with an urgent need to solve extreme low back symptoms. He has a very complex history of low back problems and pain.

His back history dates back to 1996 when he underwent an L4 – L5 microdiscectomy at Columbia Presbyterian Hospital. He did very well from the surgery and continued to do well until the 1980s when he started experiencing more back pain possibly from significant athletic activity.

Mr. Capozzi underwent a second surgery in December 2018 at the Laser Spine Institute at the L4 – L5 level.

He then underwent a third surgery at the L2 – L3 level on the right side at Bio-Spine in Tampa, Florida. This appears to have been a bilateral decompression performed only from the right side.

It appears that the first and second surgeries were successful, but after the third surgery, Mr. Capozzi began having recurrent pain in October of 2019.

His back pain is positional. It's better when he flexes forward as identified when pushing a grocery cart.

He has experienced severe pain when walking or lying in a prone position. And, has found that ice packs seem to reduce inflammation and that the pain is more in the right paraspinal area of his low back. The pain lessens when sitting or bending forward.

He has no family history of acute back issues. His physical examination identifies he is 5'8" tall and weighs 185 pounds.

On exam, he has multiple incisions. The lowest incision seems to be at the L5 – S1 level. He has two paraspinal incisions from his minimally invasive fusion at the L4 – L5 level. He has a third incision on the right side of his spine which is from an L2 – L3 hemilaminotomy. He is tender in the lumbar spine.

His X-ray shows that he has had an attempted fusion at his L4 – L5 level with an interbody graft. There is some settling of the graft seen.

The screws are in good position and there is no visual loosening of the screws. He appears to have a degenerative disc at L5 – S1. He has had a laminectomy at L2 – L3 on the right side of his spine, but I cannot tell whether there is a pars defect.

His MRI from November 2019 shows that he has a recurrent disc herniation on the right side at L2 – L3. This does show crowding of the thecal sac. At L3 – L4, where he has had no surgery, there is moderate to severe spinal stenosis. At L4 – L5 he is adequately decompressed and that is where his instrumentation is present.

Also, at the L3- L4 level there is a disc herniation on the right side just above the L3 pedicle and perhaps slightly lower than the disc space that pins the L3 nerve root severely, but the thecal sac, itself, is severely compressed as well. At the L5 – S1 level, I cannot tell whether he has ever had a laminectomy.

My impression is that Mr. Capozzi has back pain that is neurogenic, likely from the pathology at L3 – L4 but perhaps even at L2 – L3 as he does have significant disc herniation present.

Unfortunately, he will need additional surgery if he hopes to have a long-term favorable outcome. I can try injections, but do not believe non-surgical procedures will work. I also suggest another more current CT scan to see if he has a pars defect on the right where he has had his previous surgery and I need to see exactly what has happened at the L3 – L4 and whether he is fused at L4 – L5.

Unfortunately, he will need additional surgery if he hopes to have a long-term favorable outcome.

History

From my earliest memories as a young boy, I was always highly active in sports. My dad had played football in college and signed to play baseball with the New York Yankees farm team. However, he was injured playing football and hurt both his knees. This injury ruined his potential baseball career, but he did join our local volunteer fire department softball team.

Given his incredible history as a baseball player, even though he could not run very well, in almost every "at bat" he would hit a home run over the fence, so he was able to then gimp along over all the bases. He and I would play baseball almost every evening after school. With my dad's help, I even became so good at baseball that I joined the same local fire department softball team.

Playing baseball with my dad almost every day, and then playing with a group of young people in a junior league gave me self confidence that has lasted my entire life.

I would get up to bat and think. *where should I hit this next pitch ... right field, left field or center field.* I never gave thought that I would miss the ball or strike out.

As a result, I believe that positive thinking I could hit the ball helped me hit the ball. In life, if you think you can, chances are you can. If you think you can't … you're probably right.

Further, when I grew up, back "in the day," we had no cell phones, computers, video games, or even TV. So, I rode my bike and played baseball almost every day. Pre-high school, I was becoming a bit of a jock.

But I believe the origins of my serious back problems started in high school when I ran the mile in the spring and cross country in the fall. I ran every day, 360 days a year in sun, rain, and even snow. I was also on the high school wrestling team, participated in gymnastics, and started aggressively participating in martial arts. I really enjoyed gymnastics because I learned to walk on my hands and that gave me great balance which was valuable in my martial arts training.

One of my best friend's brothers was a police officer in our town. His brother had served as in the Marines, stationed in Japan for many years, where he obtained a fifth-degree black belt in martial arts. He needed someone to practice with and I gladly accepted the offer.

However, in the 60s my dad worked for the power company and our family didn't have a lot of money.

I didn't want to take out a college loan to pay for college, so I enrolled in both day school and night school, three days a week, at a leading New York City college. This enabled me to attend school on Monday, Tuesday, and Wednesday, carry a full load, and work Friday, Saturday, Sunday, and Monday to pay for school. This allowed me to carry enough credits to graduate in four years. I was very proud that I paid my way through college with zero college debt.

Across the street from my college was a men's club that contained squash courts for members. I got a job working in the locker room during my breaks between classes. It was a great job, as I could set my own hours, and, when I wasn't busy managing the laundry and locker room, I could do my homework.

One day, a member's squash guest canceled at the last moment and the member asked me to "hit" squash balls with him. I had never even held a squash racquet, much less knew what squash even was until I took this job, so I was very hesitant to hit with this member. But being a jock all my life, and in great shape at that time, I agreed to give it a try.

In about 15 minutes I started to hit a squash ball quite well, and I was able to get to the ball reasonably easy given my physical condition ... but I had no concept of court strategy.

However, after about an hour, and watching how the member played, I started to learn court strategy.   Then, to the members disbelief, I started to beat him at his own game.

Soon the word went out that the "locker kid" was a good squash player and other members started calling me to play with them. I had become the club's quasi-pro and was able to give up my locker room assignment and I then scheduled my school breaks every day, to play with members.

This was an expensive club and most of the members worked on Wall Street or were serious corporate attorneys .. and they were all quite wealthy. I was making a small fortune in tips from members. But playing squash, often with very good players, enabled me to perfect "court strategy." Little by little I became very good at squash. Once I perfected court strategy, I was even able to start playing tournaments at other clubs. Again, more stress on my back.

During our college winter breaks, I started snow skiing in Vermont. Again, because I was quite fit, I picked up snow skiing rather easily.

I continued with my interest in martial arts, but now skiing added to the beginning of stress on my back at an early age.

Following my graduation form college, I joined the military during the Vietnam War. During my military experience, and thanks to my early years in gymnastics, I held a record at my base for doing 100 one-handed push-ups and for walking 200 yards upside down on my hands. The ability to walk a great distance on my hands proved invaluable for "balance" when skiing and for martial arts. However, I also believe my activities during the Vietnam War greatly contributed to the beginnings of my back problem.

After my honorable discharge from military service. I moved to Vermont for a period to "clear my head and my stress." And, to take a job skiing on the ski patrol at Bromley Mountain in Manchester, Vermont.

I arrived at the mountain at 6:00 in the morning every day to ride to the top in a snowcat and then clear trails before the mountain opened. I skied every day for over 10 hours a day, seven days a week, and became proficient enough to become a ski instructor.

I also participated in downhill racing. Which was wonderful for my back!!! However, my life as a ski instructor was very short lived. As a new instructor, I was assigned to work with young children on the "bunny" or "beginners" slope.

Young children tended to be afraid and many just stood on the slope and wouldn't ski. Or if they did try to ski, they fell, which required me to help them to get up. Sometimes I had to hold them when they started crying for mom and dad, who were out skiing on the mountain. The parents weren't concerned because they knew they had a professional ski instructor-babysitter. These young skiers also had to go to the bathroom constantly or just wanted to drink a hot chocolate in the lodge. It was a nightmare and, because I was not moving much on the beginner's slope, I ended up getting freezing cold.

So, I quit being an instructor after one month and returned to skiing on the ski patrol. But skiing about 10 hours a day, seven days a week, over large bumps, called moguls, in the slope certainly didn't help my back either.

During this time, I continued in my martial arts training and marathon running. But as I think back to my life in Vermont, I'm convinced that aggressive skiing certainly was a factor in my life of back problems.

Then on Easter Sunday, I was making a ski movie for the mountain, and while doing a royal christie ...which requires the skier to bend one leg back and rest the other ski on his shoulder ... thus skiing on only one ski, I set the tip of that ski into a hole in the snow called a sitzmark. In the 1960's, release bindings were just coming into use, but racer didn't use them because on hard checks, the boot could "pop out" of the binding. On that day, I did not have release bindings, and I went completely over the top of the ski and broke my tibia and severely wrenched my back.

That was a wakeup call for me. I had a college education, was making $80 a week, and now had a broken leg and a damaged back. So, I applied to American Airlines at LaGuardia Airport for a job.

I was accepted by American Airlines and started in an understudy program with a goal to go into management. After three months I was promoted to supervisor ... and then to a manager at LaGuardia. I went on to become a sales rep, and then was promoted to their general office.

Over my eight years with America, I was promoted eight times and left American as a director of marketing in their corporate headquarters.

But I reached the point where my next promotion would have been vice president. With few vice president in the company, I realized that it might take perhaps five years before a position opened, so I made the decision to leave American.

In the '70s, I then joined a division of the Midland Bank Group as a vice president. At that time Midland was one of the largest international banks in the world.

Over the next five years I was promoted five times. However, I was also traveling about 25 days each month around the world. Once a month to London for board meetings. But able to travel on the Concord. I didn't like that airplane. It was like flying in a cigar tube. But it sure was fast.

In 1979 my son was born, and I didn't want a son to grow up without a dad, so I quit a wonderful job and left the division of the Midland Bank Group. Then I was its CEO of North America. I started my own company in one of the apartments in the New York townhouse that we bought. Being at home with my wife and new son was a blessing.

During this time, I had joined the New York Athletic Club and played squash as often as possible and ran in two New York City marathons.

The first company I started proved very successful and in the next few years, I started four additional companies. All did very well, and in 1981, my daughter was born.

But in 1981 my wife was diagnosed with stage-four cancer and Sloan Kettering gave her three months to live. We were devastated. My wife and I knew that it would be impossible for me to raise two babies alone in the city, so we sold our townhouse and all my companies for an obscene profit. Enough money for me to buy a large estate in Connecticut and retire at age 40. Our home in Connecticut was on 10 acres of land that had never been cleared. It contained nine acres of dense woods, areas of swamp, and poison ivy everywhere. Dangerous for young children. At the time we didn't own a car as one wasn't needed living in NYC. We took taxis everywhere, or if we left the city, we rented a car.

So, now in Connecticut, I bought a pickup truck and a backhoe because I knew I needed to make the new property safe for our children.

And retired, I hired a nurse and a nanny to help my wife and to watch the children, while I worked every day cutting trees, moving dirt to fill in the swamps, and building stone walls around the entire perimeter of the property. All work that is dangerous for someone with a bad back.

Incredibly, my wife survived without chemotherapy or radiation. She was a Christian Scientist early in her life and she had learned to meditate every day to fight the cancer.

She would meditate for hours focusing on her white cells killing the cancer. Sloan Kettering could not believe she survived, and we had several universities ask that we write a book about her experience using mind over matter. Perhaps one day we'll do that. But as I write this book, my wife of 56 years is still with me.

Then, in 1983, with my wife in remission, I went back to work, and started more companies. The first company provided sales support for a large firm that paid a huge commission. I was very successful with that firm. As a part of my commission, they gave me an enormous bonus (over a million dollars) that enabled me to build a squash court on our property. I then built a barn with my office, a gym, and the squash court in the barn. This allowed me to play squash with neighbors almost every day.

However, the property also contained a tennis court that was built by the previous owner. Growing up rather poor, my family never joined a club, so I had never even held a tennis racquet.

But everyone coming to our home thought I must be a great tennis player or else why would we have a tennis court? I didn't even own a tennis ball, so, after about a year, I hired the local town tennis pro to teach me how to play tennis. I already had a better-than-average understanding of "court strategy" from years of playing squash, and I had developed an almost perfect "eye to ball" coordination from tournament squash, so I quickly picked up tennis. After about three months of playing tennis every day, I started to beat the pro. I grew to love tennis and played it as often as I could, but that too took its toll on my back.

I had developed a killer serve, but that serve caused me to almost become addicted to Advil to help with my now constant back pain.

It was about then that I also took up golf. I joined a wonderful club in Milford, Connecticut, and I also got totally addicted to the game. I tried to play late in the afternoon because the "older golfers" played in the mornings, and usually there was no one playing late in the day. This allowed me to play with two different colored balls and in effect, play 18 holes twice at once. Golf is another sport that is dangerous to anyone with a bad back. Think about it … swinging a club as hard as you can with a twisting motion to try to hit a ball 300 yards, is just not smart.

Over the years, I also continued skiing, and when the children were old enough, we bought a home on Stratton Mountain in Vermont.

Our children had taken up skiing before they turned four, and we went to Vermont almost every Friday night in the winter with as many of their friends as possible to ski.

In 1996, while ski racing down a black diamond trail, over moguls, I herniated my L4-5 discs to the extent that it ended my skiing at that time. For about a year, I tried everything possible to prevent surgery. The pain was incredible. I visited a variety of chiropractors, yoga instructors, and even tried hanging upside down via boots attached to a bar in the ceiling for decompression. Nothing worked and my condition worsened.

Finally, my condition became so bad that I gave in and sought surgery. My research to find the right surgeon led me to a doctor who, in those years, did "inoperable brain surgery" at Columbia Presbyterian Hospital in New York City. I felt if this doctor could do brain surgery, he could certainly fix a herniated disc.

On my first visit he put my X-ray on his viewing screen and remarked: "This is one of the worst herniations I have ever seen. How are you standing the pain?"

I told him that I was taking five Advil's every four hours. He then commented: "Well, this is easy. I can either fix your back overnight or fix your stomach in a few weeks because you're going to burn a hole in it with so much Advil."

So, in 1996, I had my first surgery at Columbia Presbyterian Hospital, and it proved to be an amazing success. The following day I felt 100% better. My doctor advised me that just because I felt better I should not ski, play tennis, golf, squash, run, build more stone walls, or do anything physical for at least three months, which I certainly adhered to.

After six months, my back had healed magnificently, and I started all my "jock" activities again, including golf. My constant goal to drive a ball further, was devastating to my back. I finally had to give up golf or risk more surgery, but I continued to play tennis, squash, and run great distances. None of which was great for my back.

In 2015 we sold our home in Connecticut and moved to Nokomis, Florida. This is a small town on the Gulf of Mexico in Sarasota County.

Nokomis is an Indian name and they settled in Nokomis because Nokomis had never been hit by a hurricane in recorded history. It's why we picked this town too.

We bought a large home on a large plot of land, but the land needed work.

The builder had mortgage issues which was great for our purchase price, but he had not finished the landscaping. So, I started to improve the property. I planted over 50 palm trees, built a new sprinkler system, and put down St. Augustine sod lawns. I also continued running and even took up bicycle riding.

Everything was going well until 2018, when my back went out again primarily due to continued daily long-distance running and pounding on the highway. I was training for my third New York Marathon and running 15 miles every day. My yard landscaping work didn't help either.

So, in 2018 I went to a medical group called The Laser Spine Institute in Tampa, Florida, where they did a very small micro incision operation that corrected a new problem at my L4-L5 level. That procedure was very successful, and I stopped almost all exercise for the next five months, including aggressive yard work. Then in 2019, I had started running again, bike riding and yard work, and my back went out again.

Following my surgery in 2018, The Laser Spine Institute had gone out of business, which was a shame, because they ran a wonderful facility. I continued my research and found Bio-Spine, also located in Tampa. I had a third "micro-surgery" back procedure at my L2-L3 level at Bio-Spine. But that surgery didn't work, and my pain continued. However, with support from products such as Aleve, I could stand the pain and only lost some of my mobility.

Over the next few months, even though I had totally stopped running, squash, tennis, martial arts, golf, and aggressive yard work, my back continued to get worse, and the pain became unbearable. Quite frankly, my core became weaker from my lack of exercise and my mobility was reduced to almost nothing. I also started to gain weight from a lack of caloric burn from zero exercise.

I realized that with almost no exercise, atrophy was also setting in. Further, I started to become depressed. I tried to watch television, but that got old very quickly.

I reached a point where I couldn't sleep lying down as it caused extreme nerve pain in my legs. As such, I started sleeping in a chair because the pain was less severe while I was sitting. I slept in a chair for three months.

It got so bad that I couldn't walk to our mailbox, which is about 75 yards from my front door. If I did make it to the mailbox, I had to sit on the sidewalk to regain enough strength to just get home. One day I had a neighbor run over to help me when she saw me sitting on the sidewalk. She thought I had either fallen or had a heart attack.

If I got to the mailbox, I had to sit down on the sidewalk to regain enough strength to just get home.

Yes, it was very embarrassing to see a grown man sitting on the sidewalk, reading his mail. But having tried micro/laser surgery that didn't work, I didn't want to do that again. I knew I had to do something as I realized that a wheelchair might be in my future.

As much as I didn't want more surgery, I also knew that it might be my only course of action to save my life.   Once more I began research to find another solution using more conventional and traditional orthopedic surgeons. This research led me to three of the most highly respected orthopedic surgeons in America. They all reviewed my MRIs and X-rays, and all came to the identical conclusion: I needed a fusion.

All three said I would need a titanium plate screwed to two of my vertebrae via six large titanium screws. The cost would be over $100,000. The suggested operation would require a six- to eight-inch incision in my back, with two surgeons working together: one to hold the plate and the other to attach six screws into my spine.

The operation would take about eight hours, with a huge incision, and would require about a year of recuperation wearing an enormous brace. I would only be allowed to lift five pounds of weight during the almost 12-month recovery.

Then the concerns started. My primary physician, who believes surgery is necessary in many cases, was deeply concerned that at my age, eight hours of anesthesia could be very dangerous. While he agreed with what the three back surgeons told me based upon their reviews: he told me there was no guarantee that the surgery would even work.

It was further suggested by others that it might cause me to become paralyzed since it was such an extensive procedure. My physician considered pain medication but did not want to start me on opioids for fear I might become addicted and might never get off such strong medication. He suggested Aleve several times a day to help reduce the inflammation and pain.

My fear was that even with the surgery, I might never recover sufficiently enough to have any meaningful quality of life. So, I continued my research to explore other alternatives. This is when a former Army physical therapist, who has worked with disabled veterans in the Middle East, suggested aqua therapy. I knew nothing about aqua therapy, but I studied it extensively and consulted with a variety of experts.

After significant research, I began to believe it was something I should take very seriously, and at least try, because being weightless in a pool might not cause stress to my back, and as such there would be no significant downside.

I learned that in the pool, I could exercise my legs, arms, chest, and stomach with no stress to my back. I could also control the amount of pressure with each exercise by either increasing or decreasing the resistance or movement in the water. We have a pool in our home in Florida that is heated to 85 degrees. So even in the winter months in Florida when the temperature dropped to the 40s, I could still use the pool. Getting in and out of the pool with a 40-degree temperature was a bit daunting, but I could get back into the master bedroom quickly.

Now the thought of creating and aqua therapy program looked even more interesting. It became evident that by strengthening my core and all the muscles supporting my spine, as well as stretching many of the ligaments supporting my back, it might be possible to reduce my pain to at least a point where I might be able to sleep in my bed again. I also felt that such a program could also stop the atrophy that was becoming noticeable.

It took several weeks for me to create the exercises in this book.

Most exercises represent my desire to strengthen my core and hopefully bring more support to my spine, as well as to reduce the pain. But, as you will read, I added a few other water exercises to strengthen my arms, chest, and legs to also prevent atrophy. My thought in expanding the range of exercises I was using is that nothing I researched proved negative to having full body exercises in water. Quite the contrary. By exercising areas such as my legs via "jogging" in water, I noticed that my buttocks became much firmer, and that area of my body added additional support to my back. However, jogging in water creates no "pounding" on the spine, since I am almost totally weightless in the water. The jogging further helped my ankles, calves, and thighs.

Forward arm pulls strengthen my upper back muscles. Reverse arm pulls strengthen my chest muscles. Aqua sit-ups that are identified further in this book strengthen my stomach muscles.

The results of my program are nothing short of amazing. I do about one hour of aqua therapy each day in our pool...every day. If I jog a long distance in the water, sometimes I am in the pool for over an hour. Over the course of my program, I have only missed three days of Aqua therapy since I started the program.

I'm in my pool when it rains, during thunderstorms, and in the summer when it's very hot.

Hey, who cares if it's raining when you're in a pool.

I became totally addicted to my aqua therapy program as my back pain and mobility started to improve significantly. As I write this book, I am about 95% free of all pain. More importantly, I can sleep in my bed again, ride my bike 15 miles twice a week, work in my yard, and walk a great distance. And of interest, I am starting to stand straight again. For a long time, I was bent forward and only felt good pushing a grocery cart, as that action caused me to lean forward, and leaning on the cart helped take the pressure off my spine. I started joking with people that I was bent forward while walking because I was looking for quarters and other change on the ground to pay for my obscene lifestyle!

I know I'll never jog or run marathons again for fear that the pounding on the street will damage my back. Jogging in a pool, however, greatly reduces pounding on my spine.

I began aqua jogging for only a minute or two with very few steps, but over the course of a year, I have expanded my aqua jogging distance to over two miles each day. I use the number of steps jogged to calculate my distance.

One of my neighbors used my program, and was an Olympic swim team coach, and he recommended water weights for my ankles for greater stability in the pool and for a variety of other reasons, including assisting muscle development. So, I started wearing 2.5-pound ankle weights on each ankle for greater stability in the water and to give me a bit more weight to help strengthen my leg muscles and stomach.

However, after a few months my strength improved greatly, so I moved to five-pound weights on each ankle. You might think that 5-pound weight on your ankles is excessive, but trust me, in the pool, where you are very buoyant, you hardly notice the weights. As you read further, you will also learn that the weights are of critical importance to the program as they are essential for greater stability in the water.

I've further mentioned the weights in the equipment section.

With respect to the program, I initially started doing about 10 repetitions of each exercise you'll find in this book.

I moved slowly and cautiously at first, as I certainly didn't want to create any additional injury to my back. But, gradually, I started to increase my repetitions because I started to feel stronger. After about a year, I was doing 75—100 repetitions for each exercise.

I noticed that when I pulled the water with my arms very hard, it intensified the exercises. Plus, I found that if I "cupped" my hands during those exercises that require arm movements, it provided greater water resistance and made those exercises harder. Just moving my arms or legs through the water easily will not help me build greater fitness.

Harder work is what is needed to build greater core strength. While I found almost immediate relief from pain once I started working in the pool, it took a few months of "everyday" pool work for me to notice a vast improvement in my back condition. Again, as I write this book, I have become totally addicted to my routine and have a fear of regression if I miss a day.

If I didn't have a pool in my home and wanted to try aqua therapy, I would have considered getting a membership in a club or a place such as the YMCA where a pool is available.

All the exercises in this book can be conducted in a very small space in a pool in about four or five feet of water, so using a commercial pool should not interfere with those people who are swimming laps. Many commercial pools have special areas that are not designed for swimmers doing laps.

Now that I have arrived at a point where my back is significantly better and my quality of life is incredibly better, I again work in the yard, ride my bike twice a week, and have no problem walking great distances. However, I do wear my back brace when doing yard work or doing anything that might cause stress to my back, just for added insurance.

The bottom line is that aqua therapy has given me my life back. It has not only helped my back, but it has also given back my stomach abs, allowed me to lose about 18 pounds of weight, which is great for core and back strength, and I can once again sleep in a bed at night.

Most importantly, I am taking absolutely no prescription or over-the-counter meds.

Another lesson I learned is that "surgeons suggest surgery." It's what they studied in school and it's what they do for a living; in my case, as you will read, I found it very worthwhile to explore other, non-surgical solutions.

Equipment Needed

Exercising in a swimming pool can be an amazing experience because you will be "weightless." Being weightless greatly reduces stress on your back and lessens the potential for harm during workouts. However, one negative of exercising in a pool is that I tended to "float around" and, without stability, most of the exercises identified in this book will not be as effective as they could be.

Fortunately, the solution was easy: I use aqua ankle weights on both my ankles to "ground" my feet to the bottom of the pool and to give me fantastic additional stability.

As you will read on the following page, I also use a small surfboard, sometimes called a "boogie board" or "float board." Yes, the same one that young people use at the beach. Why use such a board?

Because it allows me to do a variety of exercises using my legs and stomach that would normally be almost impossible to accomplish without this tool.

Again, this is like what young people use at the beach. The best size is 36" x 16" wide. At the beach, the board is usually held in a vertical position, with your hands on each side.

A small float board:

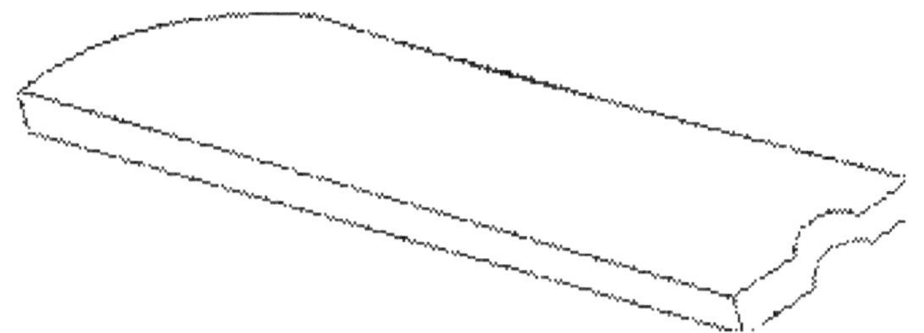

However, when I am using it for aqua therapy, I found that it's best to hold the board horizontally with my hands at each side of the lower corner as shown in the illustration below. The reason why I hold the board at each "lower" corner is that I need to use more stomach muscles to accomplish the exercises I'm about to describe.

If I try holding the board in other positions, I notice that it takes less stomach effort to do the exercises, but building my core to protect my back requires very strong stomach muscles.

Ankle water weights:

These are vital for greater stability in the water and for increased strength building. As already mentioned, I started with 2.5-pound weights for each ankle however, I quickly learned that since I was weightless in the pool, it would be better to use heavier weights. So, I switched to five-pound weights for each ankle. It was almost impossible to notice the difference between the lighter and heavier weights in the water.

Ankle aqua weights can be purchased in a variety of retail stores that sell pool equipment and can be found on Amazon or via Google. Ask for ankle weights that can be used in a pool. I found that it was almost impossible to do most of the exercises in this book without them.

OVER THE PAST ALMOST THREE YEARS I HAVE ONLY MISSED THREE DAYS WHERE I HAVE NOT DONE MY AQUA THERAPY. IF YOU START THIS PROGRAM, DON'T EXPECT GREAT RESULTS IF YOU DON'T DO YOUR EXERCISES RELIGIOUSLY. EVEN CREATE A "SHORT" PROGRAM FOR WHEN YOU HAVE LIMITED TIME.

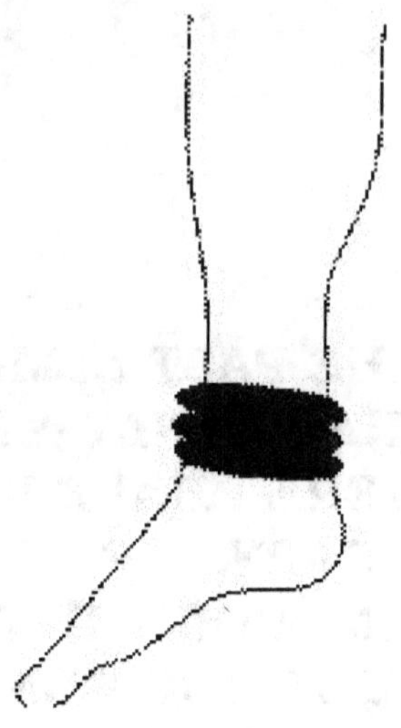

Ankle Weights

The Exercises

1. Leg and Stomach Exercise

This exercise will strengthen and help legs, abdominal muscles, and core. It also helps relieve stiffness in your joints.

Actions:

1. Hold your float board lengthwise with arms extended to the far lower corners of your board.

2. Wear your ankle weights.

3. Keep your legs perfectly straight and lift each leg straight up until you can see your toes on the other side of the board and out of the water.

4. Pull in your stomach to help build your stomach muscles.

Start doing only 20 reps with each leg. Then graduate to more reps as your legs and stomach get stronger. Set a goal to do perhaps 100 leg lifts as you developed more strength. When I started to feel a burning sensation in my stomach muscles that was a good thing. It meant that this exercise was working. My stomach was getting stronger, and strong abdominals are critical for greater core strength … and a better back.

Hold the board so your legs and knees can
go under it.

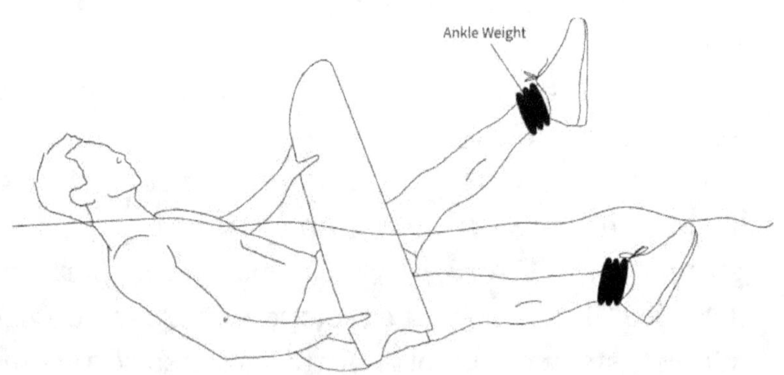

As I write this book, my stomach muscles have gotten rock hard. One day I approached our 17-year-old yard helper who comes on the weekends to help with weeding, mulch, and general yard cleanup. I told him about my aqua therapy program and mentioned that my stomach muscles had improved greatly. Then I asked him to punch me in the stomach. He initially refused. But on insistence he gave me a weak punch. I laughed and said: "Is that the best you got?" So, he punched me harder. I laughed again and called him a name that I can't put in this book. That upset him to the point where he hauled off and gave me a punch so hard that he hurt his wrist.

His punch bounded off my stomach to his total amazement. Prior to my aqua therapy program, that punch would have taken the wind out of my body, and I would have been on the ground.

Over the two years that I have been doing my program every day, I've noticed that my chest, arms, and legs have developed new muscles to go along with my new "six-pack."

2. Leg, Stomach, and Hamstring Exercise

This exercise does not use the float board but does use the ankle weights. It requires I hold on to the edge of my pool with both hands.

Actions:

1. Facing the edge of my pool in water that is about three feet deep, hold on to the edge of the pool with both hands.

2. Always use ankle weights.

3. Bring your left knee up in front towards the wall, but then continue to bring it up towards your chest as high as you can. Then bring it back down.

4. Continue by extending your left leg straight back behind as high and as far as you can. This will stretch your hip flexors and build your stomach and core muscles. It adds improvement to your hamstrings, which are so important to your back health.

5. Hold your leg straight behind for two or three seconds with your weights on. Pull your stomach in, as that will help you build core an abdominal muscle.

6. When I started this program, I tried to do 15 to 20 repetitions, and then switched legs. As I write this book, I am doing 100 reps. However, I know never to do more repetitions of any exercise beyond what feels comfortable to me.

NEVER PUSH EXERCISES SUCH AS A STRETCH OF YOUR HAMSTRINGS. STRETCH ONLY A LITTLE EACH TIME YOU ARE IN THE POOL. IF YOU OVER STRETCH YOUR HAMSTRINGS, YOU COULD INJURE THEM AND IT WILL TAKE WEEKS OR EVEN MONTHS TO HEAL DON'T RUSH YOUR AQUA THERAPY PROGRAM FOR ANY EXERCISES. YOUR BODY WILL TELL YOU YOUR LIMITS. CONSTANT EXERCISE WITH MODERATE EFFORT IS MUCH BETTER THAN TRYING TO OBTAIN QUICK RESULTS.

Exercise 2: Leg, stomach, and hamstring exercise

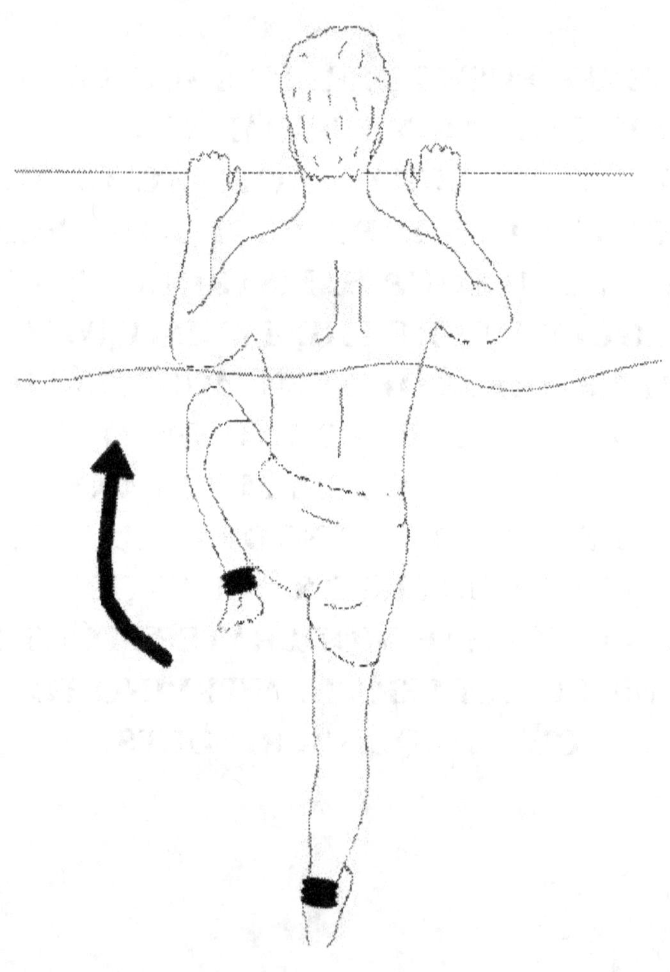

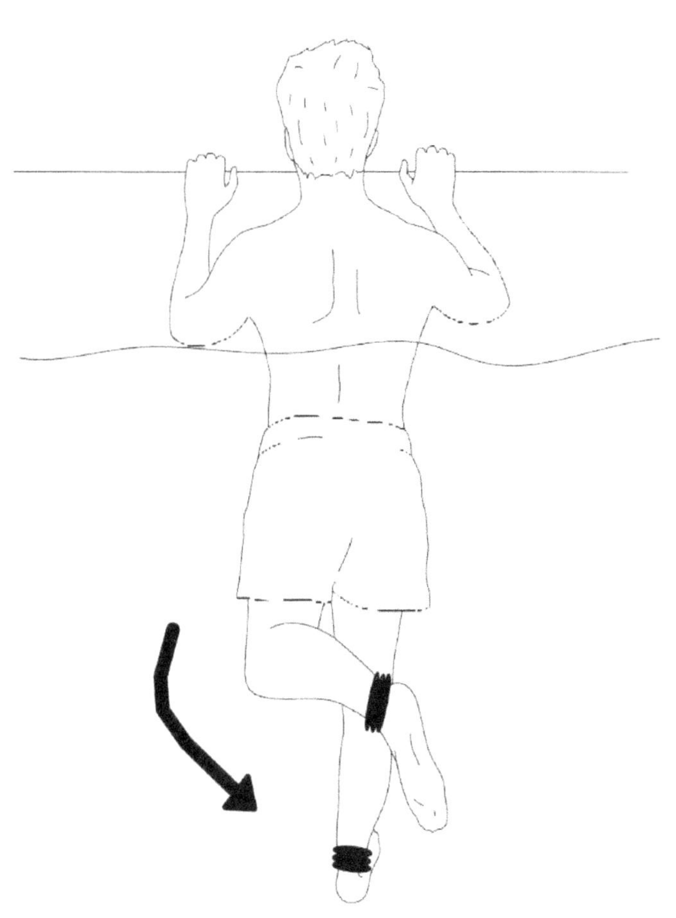

3. Hip Exercise

This exercise helped build my core and strengthen the muscles and ligaments around my hips.

Actions:

1. Still without using your board, hold on to the side of the pool with both hands in about three feet of water.

2. Have your ankle weights on.

3. Bring your left leg straight out to one side (90 degrees) and raise it in the water as high as you can, then bring it back down. My long-term goal was to get my toes out of the water. As I first started aqua therapy, I could only raise my foot about as high as my knee. Years ago, I could bring my leg up to almost my shoulder, but I suspect that by not doing any stretching for several years it causes atrophy and a loss of movement. As I write this book, I can now just get my toes completely out of the water.

4. When I started this exercise, I also tried to do 20 of these movements. However, as I increased my strength, I eventually achieved 50 reps on a regular basis.

5.Then switch legs. Do the same with your right leg and lift it up 90 degrees to get your toes out of the water.

6 Now bring each leg forward, but not perfectly straight. Bring one leg off to the left side and the other off to the right side. The trick is to stretch the sides of your body and as you lift your leg forward and then pull it to the side, you will feel the pull in your hips.

7.Next, try to lift each leg straight back to the rear. Then move it back but to the left so that you can feel a pull on your side. Do 20 reps and they switch lets and pull the other leg back but to the right side.

By moving your leg lifts from positions 90 degrees out to each side, then doing the exercise with your leg a bit forward, and then a bit to the back and off to each side a bit, you're using a range of muscles all around your hips as well as our lower back to assist in strengthening your core. Here is where something very interesting happened to me.

I honestly don't know exactly what exercise has helped my back the most. So, each day I do all of them.

But, when I first started and I lifted my left leg back but off to the side a bit, I saw stars. It really hurt. Lifting it straight back but not off to the side was totally okay. So, I concentrated on the lift that hurt me so much. I started out doing only about three repetitions and did so very slowly due to the pain.

Each day when I got to this exercise, I tried to increase the repetitions and hold my leg back and a bit to the side longer, with my weights on After about three months, the pain diminished considerably, and I started to do more repetitions.

The same exercise on my right side created no pain, so I knew that something was wrong on my left side.

About six months into the program, the pain on my left side had completely gone away, and it was the first time that I really knew that I was doing something great as the overall condition of my back had improved so much. This is when I started to walk much greater distances with much less pain.

While I had noticed improvement after three months, it was nothing like the improvement once I was able to advance this one exercise.

An initial goal was to get my toes out of the water with each lift. That did not happen right away, but after a few months I was able to stretch my muscles and ligaments so that I can get my legs high enough to see my toes out of the water.

I pull in my stomach with each leg lift. And I try to concentrate to take a deep breath with each movement. Keep in mind that there are muscles inside your body that support your organs, and it is important to strengthen them too.

REMEMBER, IN ALL THE EXERCISES WHERE YOU NEED TO KEEP YOUR ANKLES UP HIGH AT THE TOP OF THE WATER, THESE EXERCISES BUILD STOMACH MUSCLES. YOUR WEIGHTS CAUSE ISOMETRIC ACTIVITY AS IT IS YOUR STOMACHH MUSCLES THAT ARE HOLDING YOUR LEGS UP HIGH IN THE WATER.

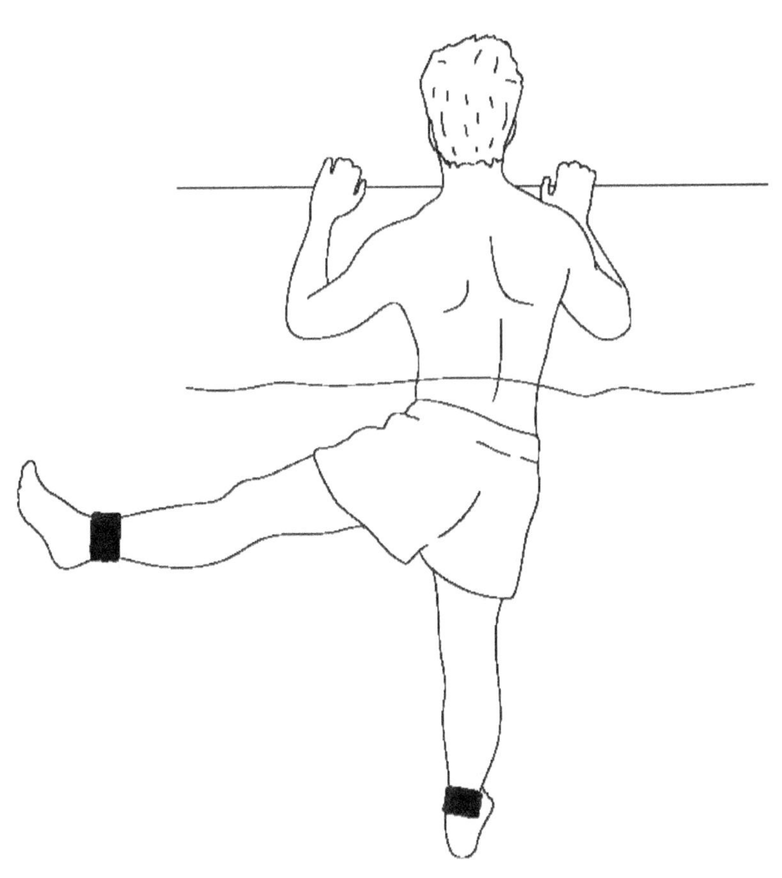

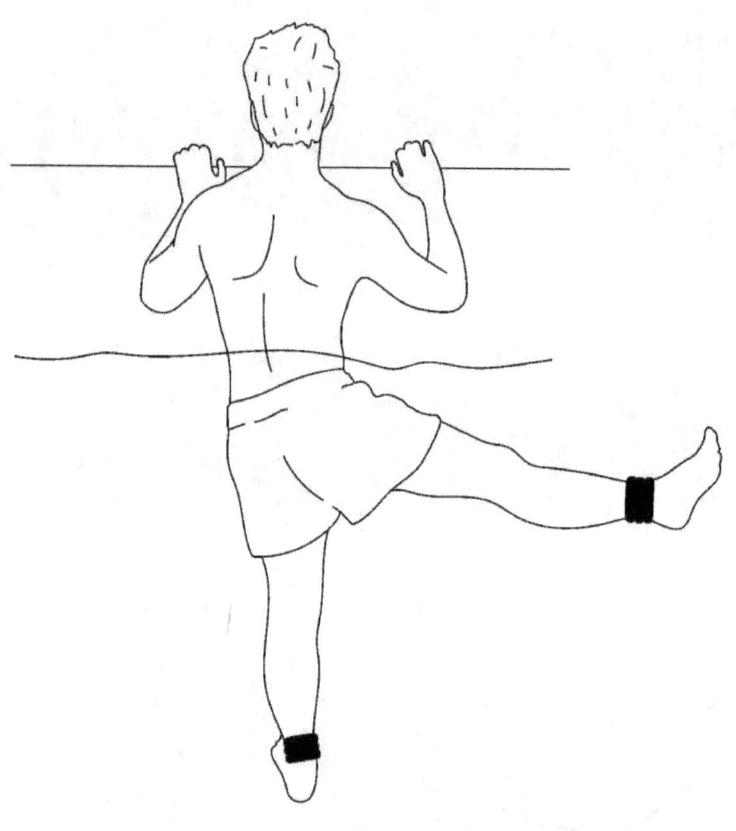

4. Arms Forward

This exercise helped build my chest, upper back, arms, and stomach.

Actions:
1. Stand in neck- or shoulder-high water.

2. Wear ankle weights for greater stability.

3. Bend your knees a bit if you're in the shallow end so that the water level is about as high as your shoulders. By bending your knees, a little bit, your also take stress off your lower back.

4. Bring your arms forward straight out in front, and never lock your elbows.

5. With your arms straight and fully extended, cup your hands for maximum water resistance.

6. "Pull" your arms horizontally from the front along each side of your body ... as far back behind as possible and comfortable, keeping them perfectly straight but not locked.

7. Try use your feet to keep your body straight in an upright position. Pulling your arms back will cause you to move forward. Try to not do that.

Using your feet to help with stability will also allow you to pull harder. Remember to always cup your hands for greater resistance. Each week increase the effort to pull the water ... harder and harder. The harder you pull, the more you'll get out of this exercise.

If you simply move your arms slowly through the water, you might get clean, but you'll not get any value out of this exercise. This exercise will build your upper back muscles. Try to initially do 20 reps with each movement. Set a goal to do at least 50 reps.   But keep pulling as hard as you can.   That's how you'll build strength.

With the front pull, try to also pull your stomach in and keep your abdominals contracted. Pulling in your stomach and contracting your abdominals help build stronger abs and adds more core strength, which helps support the spine.

As with all these exercises, try to not forget to breathe deep with each pull. Again, deep breathing helps the muscles supporting your lungs and keeps oxygenated and in turn helps add to a stronger core.

After about a month I started to see that my upper back, arm, and chest muscles got harder.

I knew that if I overdid this exercise, I might feel muscle soreness in my chest muscles the next day, but that is not a bad thing. In fact, muscle soreness following any exercise means that I am breaking down the muscle and it will then heal stronger. If I did get muscular discomfort the following day, I do not do this exercise for at least a day and then, when I felt better, I continue my program. To potentially avoid muscle stress, start slowly and built reps over time.

Start with arms forward

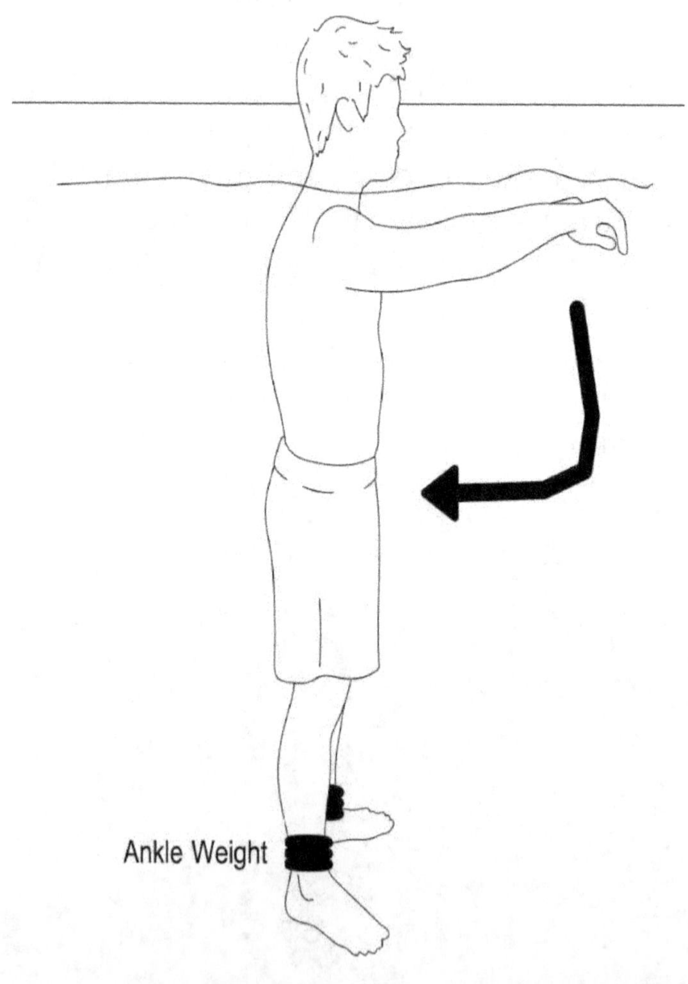

Pull arms back as far as possible.

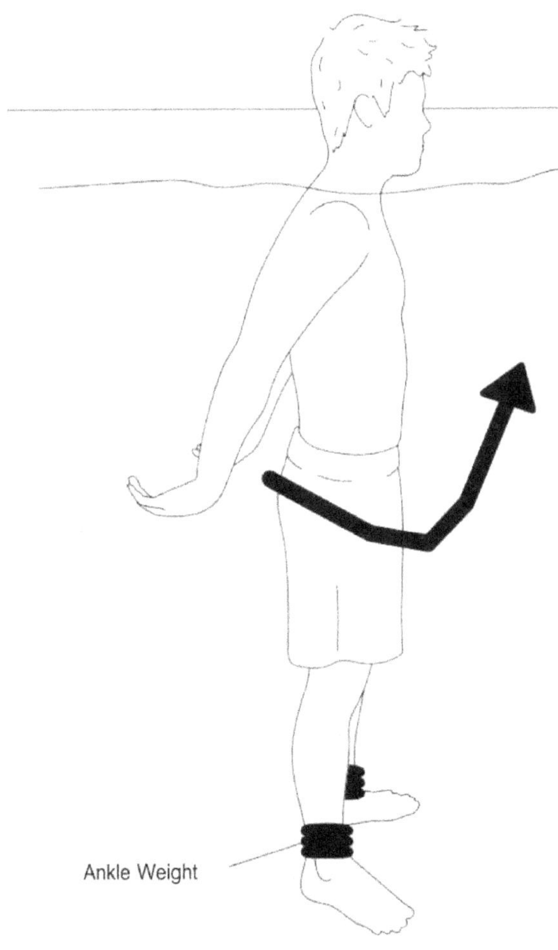

5.   Arms Back

This exercise helps build your upper back, chest, arms, and stomach.

Actions:

1.   Stand neck or shoulder high in our pool. If in shallow water, bend your knees a bit to lower your body so that your arms are parallel with the top of the water.

2. Have your ankle weights on for greater stability.

3. Pull in your stomach.

4. Breathe deeply with each pull.

5. With your arms straight but not locked, extend them back behind you as far as possible. It's important to keep your arms perfectly straight and then pull them forward with your hands cupped for greater resistance.

You should feel the impact on your upper back, and chest ... but it also strengthens your core.

If you have an added goal of building biceps and triceps, then exercises #4 and #5 will help do it. For biceps, bring your arms down to your sides and then with hands cupped, put them up hard just like you'd do with a barbell. The reverse is what you do to build triceps and forearm muscles. From the top of the water, cup your hands, and pull your arms down to your sides.

Of interest, when I first started aqua therapy, I had what the doctors called "trigger fingers" and a tingling in the tips of my fingers. It's called carpal tunnel syndrome. A few of my 10 fingers would lock in a bent position and I would have to manually pull them forward to unlock them. This is said to be caused by a pinched nerve in the wrist. My doctors told me that this condition could be cured with surgery. However, after about three months of doing exercises #4 and #5, all my fingers returned to normal. Obviously, I did not have surgery and I have done nothing to improve this condition other than exercises #4 and #5

Arms Back

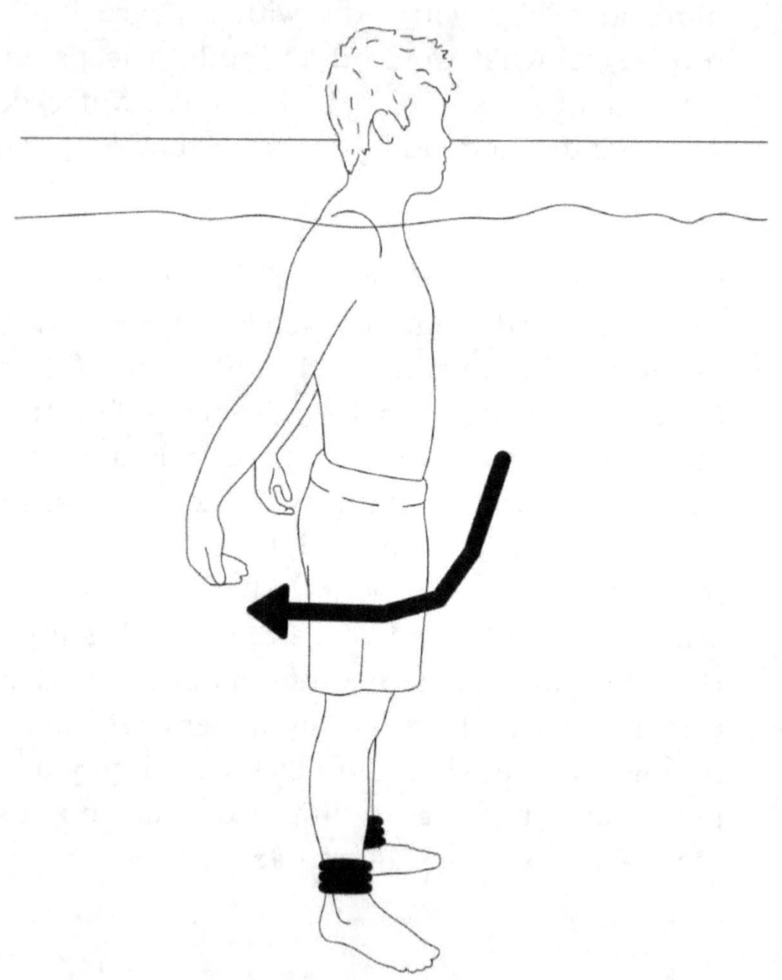

Arms Forward

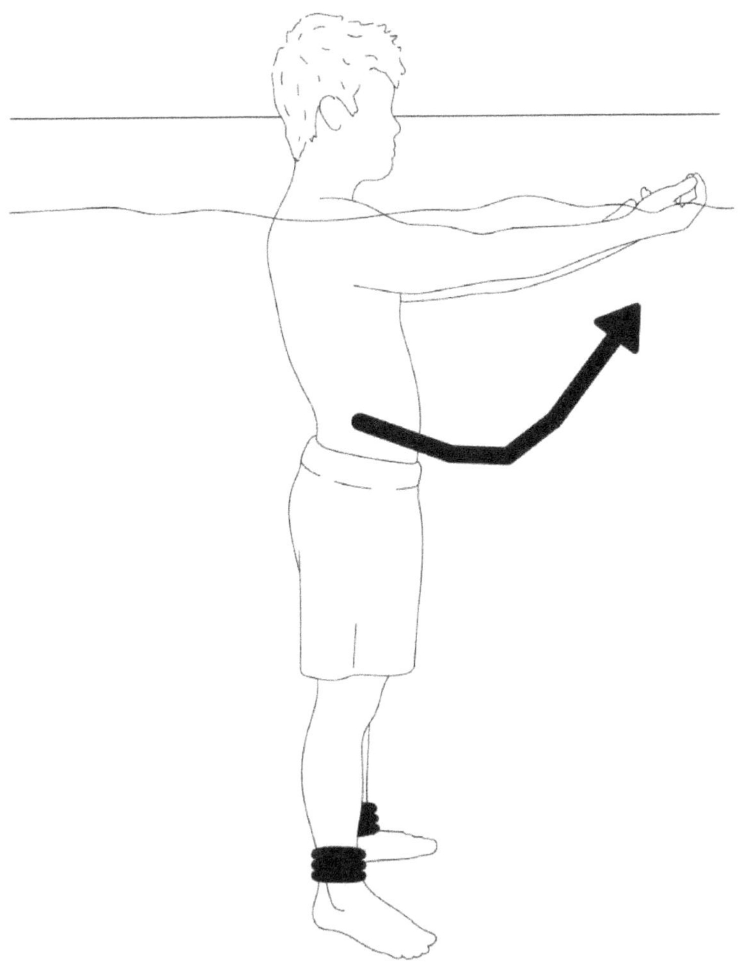

6. Jogging

This exercise helped build the core, upper thighs, calf muscles and glutes. It also strengthened lungs if you deep breath.

1.Hold the float board "horizontally" and not "vertically" for stability while standing in waist-high water.

2.Wear ankle weights.

3. Start running slowly to loosen up. Run in place and try to bring your knees up just a bit, but not as high as possible. You only need to bring each foot up about 6 to 8 inches.

4. Contract your abdominals.

5. Breathe deeply with each step.

6. Start by counting each time your right foot leaves the ground. Start with 25 steps and built more steps over time.

7. Stand upright and hold the board in a way that enables you to be straight as you jog. When I first started, I was bending forward when I walked. Now I'm still standing a bit forward, but I'm standing much straighter.

I cannot tell you how much I miss long-distance running and marathons. But jogging in the pool is as close to jogging on the street as I have found. Plus, in the pool I'm "weightless" and pool jogging causes little to no stress on my back.

Also, after I had done this exercise for several weeks, I increased the number of steps and the speed. As I write this book, I am jogging about two miles each day, and I've seen a major hardening of my stomach and glutes.

Here's another suggestion ... if you have a spouse, buy two sets of weight and two float boards. Then plan you day with your spouse to both do aqua therapy together. This program can be done early in the morning or late in the afternoon. My pool has lights, so I have even done my exercises after dark.

Jogging

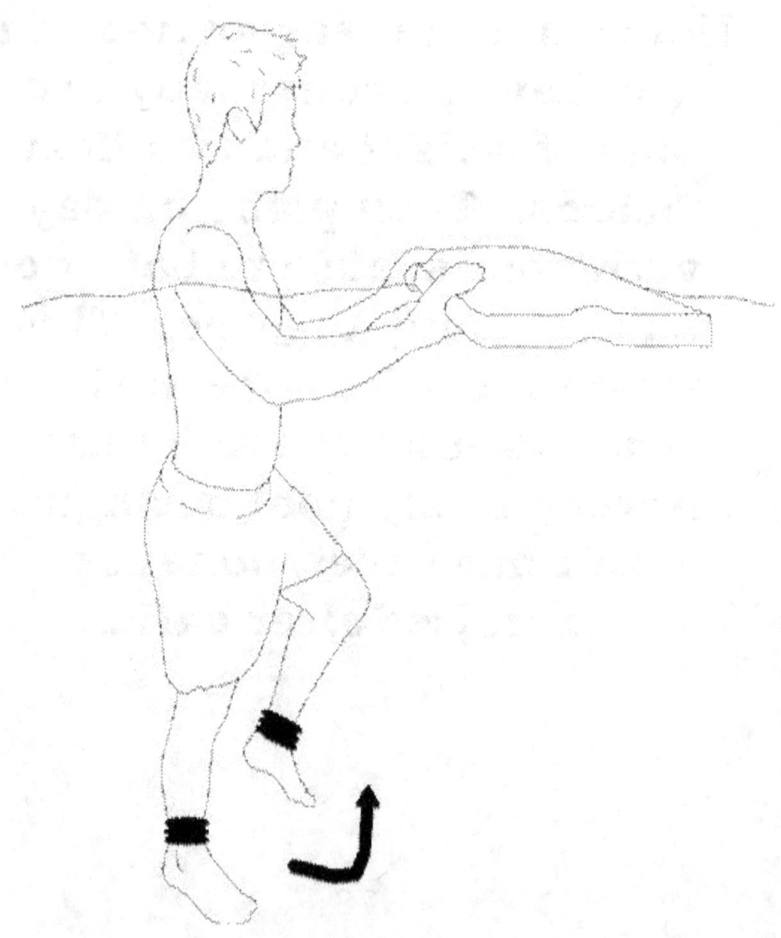

7. Frog Kick

This exercise assists in core and stomach development and strengthened the hips.

Actions:

1. Facing forward, hold your board horizontally via the lower corners of each side.

2. Wear ankle weights.

3. Extend your legs forward as high as possible in the water.

4. Open or spread each as far as possible.

5. Keep your feet at the surface of the water and your legs straight as possible.

6. Then bring your legs together quickly with a scissor-kick movement. Don't just bring your leg together easily, pull them hard. The harder the better.

7. Pull in your stomach when doing this exercise.

8. Don't forget to breathe.

I started with 20 reps and set a goal to do at least 50 reps each time I did my workout.

As mentioned earlier, by keeping your toes at the top of the water with your ankle weight on.

You're doing isometrics that are building your stomach muscles. It's your stomach muscles that are holding your feet to the top of the water. And this will build your six-pack.

Again … this program was designed by me with a lot of thought as to what my goal was. Sure, I wanted to support my back, but I also wanted to build my arms, legs, shoulders, and neck. The readers of this book need to do the same thing I did. Create your own program based upon your needs. But again, be sure to have your primary physician review your program to ensure you will not be doing something that might not be best for you.

Frog Kick

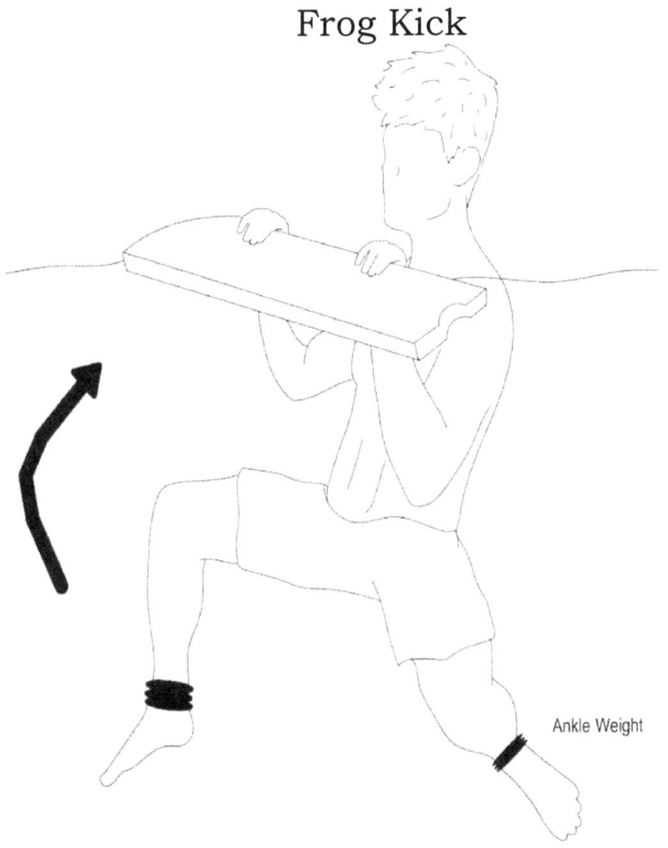

8. Hamstring Stretch

This exercise will stretch the hamstrings, which are very important in reducing back pain.

Actions:

1. At the entry steps of the pool, extend a leg straight out with your toes on the step.

2. Try to keep your back straight.

3. Then bend or hinge forward until you can feel a stretch in your hamstring and calf muscle.

4. Pull in your stomach.

5. Don't forget to breathe.

6. Hold that "pull and stretch" for about five seconds and then move back up and switch legs.

7. Repeat this exercise several times, but be careful not to stretch too hard. You don't want to hurt the hamstring.

The hamstrings are of critical importance to your back health. If you do not stretch them, they'll pull downwards and that impacts your lower back.

If you're not infirmed, you can work on your hamstrings on land, and there are dozens of books you can buy that will give you instructions as to how to exercise your hamstrings.   However, in the water it's very easy to do..

However, be very careful to not stretch to hard as you can easily hurt your hamstrings. If you do that, it could take weeks or even months for them to heal.

When I first started, I did about 20 stretches with my left leg and then switched legs. As I advanced, I tried to increase these stretches from five seconds to at least 20 seconds for each leg. My goal was to get to a point where I could put my chin down and touch my knee.

Hamstring stretch

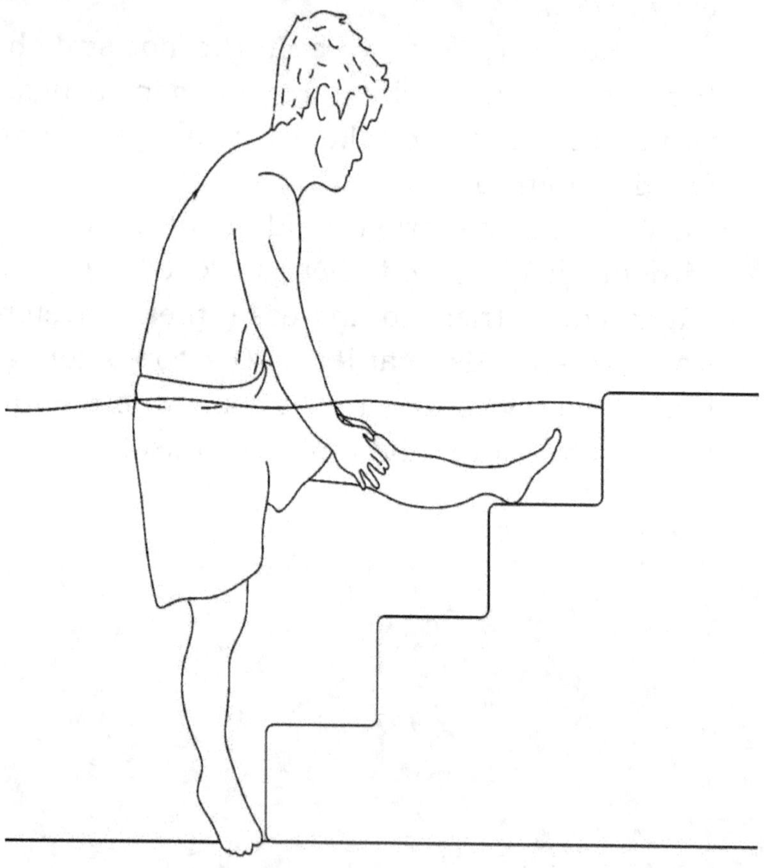

9. Abdominal Crunch

This exercise strengthened stomach muscles.

I think this exercise is one of the most important in this entire book. I mentioned earlier the abdominals are so important to good back health that I am mentioning them again.

Your goal should be to obtain a six-pact that you would be proud to bring to a beach. That six-pack will help your back enormously.

Actions:

1. Wear leg weights.

2. Hold the board horizontally and not vertically, with your grip at the lower right and left corners.

3. Exhaling, bring both knees under the board toward your chest.

4. The trick to making this exercise easier is to bring your arms, while holding your board at the lower right and left corners, forward and perfectly straight as you move my knees up to your chest. Try to keep your board flat in the water and as far out in front of you as possible. This enables you to bring your knees closer to your chest more easily.

5. Without bumping your knees against the board each time you bring them under the board.

6. Again, bring your knees up as close to your chest as possible.

7.When you return your legs back straight forward and under your board, try to keep your ankles as high in the water as possible. Keeping your ankles at the top of the water while wearing leg weights requires that you use your stomach muscles to hold them in that position. This is a form of isometrics and isometrics build muscles. Lastly, as you do this exercise, send you legs back under the board slowly.

Start with only about 20 repetitions, but then increase your repetitions each day. Set a goal of at least 100 repetitions to be achieved over time. As you increased repetitions, if you start to feel a burning sensation in your stomach muscles, this is a very good thing. It means that the exercise is working, and you are building stronger stomach muscles.

In my case, after two years of doing Aqua Therapy every day, I have a stomach like a rock ... and so can you.

Abdominal Crunch

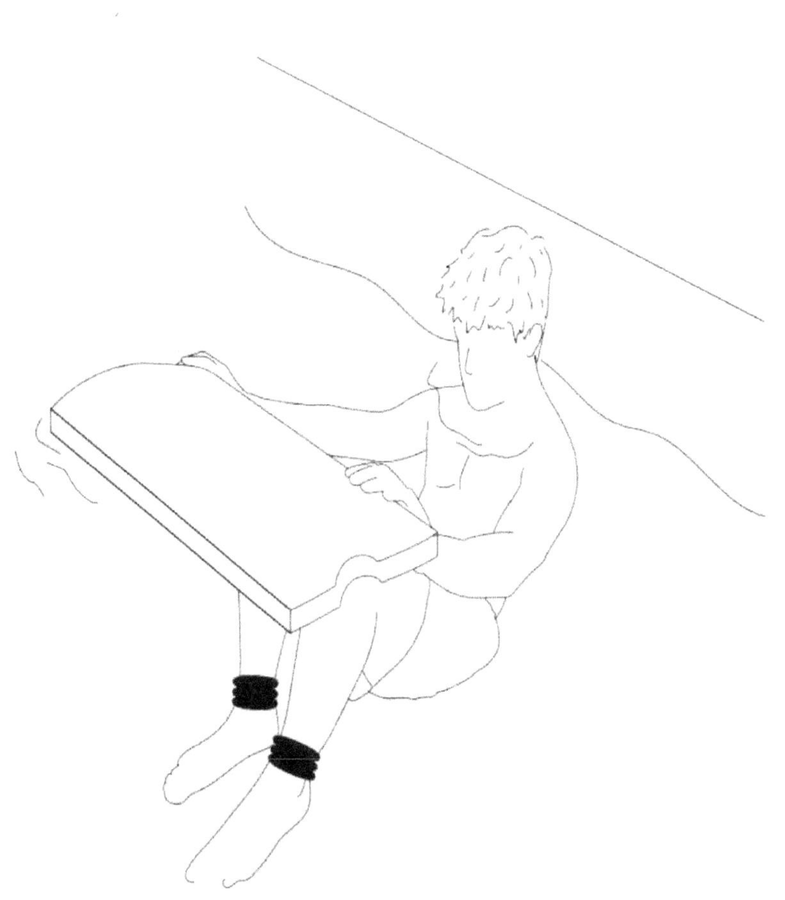

10. Decompress

This exercise can help you decompress or stretch each of the discs in your back, and reduce any pressure on any one disc.

Unfortunately, you need a pool with a "deep end".   Deep enough for your legs to not touch the bottom. However, it's possible that in a pool that is not over your head but is over five feet deep that you can decompress by bending your legs as you hang on your board.

Actions:

1. Hold your float board in any comfortable position.

2. Wear ankle weights.

3. Move to the deep end of the pool so that your legs hang straight down and don't touch the bottom of the pool.

4. Relax and hang in this position for a few minutes. The ankle weights help decompress your spine.

5. Be sure to breath in and out deeply to stretch your lungs.

DECOMPRESS

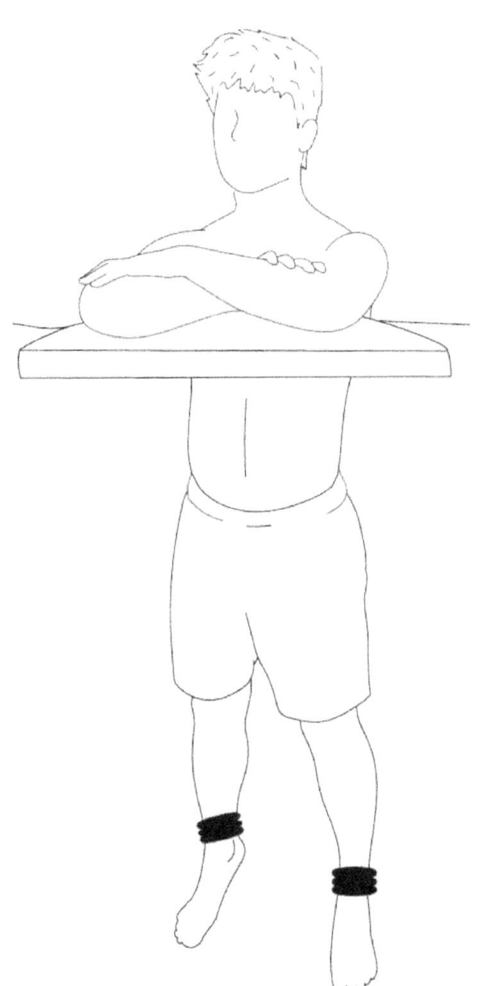

11. Side Muscles

This exercise strengthened the muscles on each side of the body. It also can strengthen stomach muscles and your core.

Actions:

1. Repeat exercise #9 above. But instead of bringing BOTH knees under the board and up to your chest, only pull ONE knee up under the board to your chest. Then switch knees and pull the other one up and under the board.

2. Wear ankle weights.

3. Try to push the board forward while keeping it flat. This allows your knee to clear the board and not bump it as you bring it under the board.

4. First bring your left knee under the board to your chest and straighten it; then bring your right knee under the board and straighten it.

5. Keep your legs and ankles as high in the water as possible.

6. Concentrate on breathing deeply as you bring each knee to your chest separately.

SIDE MUSCLES

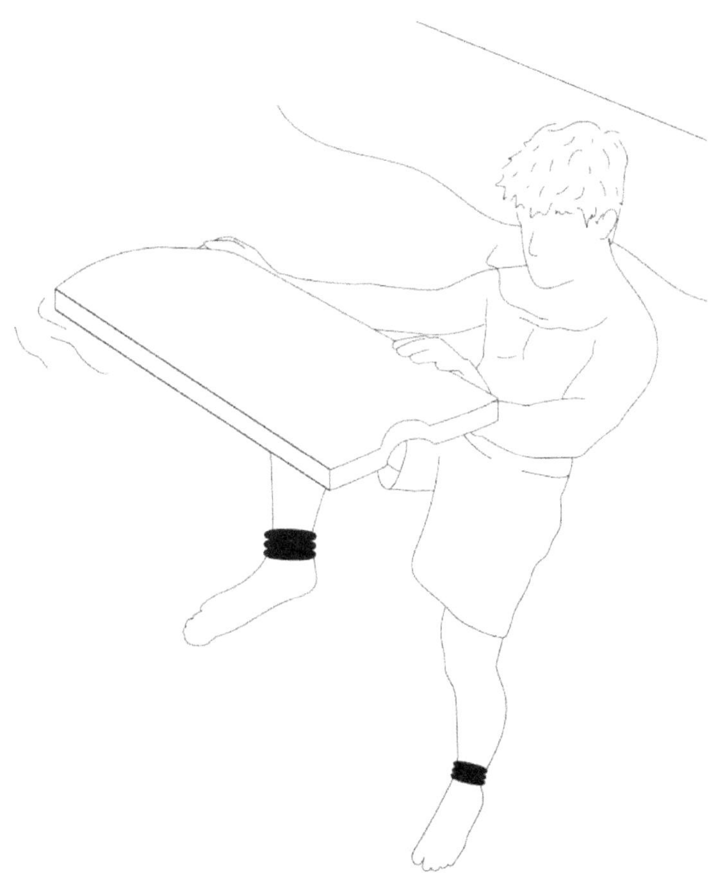

12. Calf Raises

This exercise stretches and strengthens your calf muscles. It does not focus primarily on your core, but simply being in the pool and doing these calf raises does help support total body improvement, and to those who are using aqua therapy for prevention of atrophy.

Most importantly, it's a critical exercise for those trying to prevent atrophy.

Actions:
1. Stand in about three feet of water.
2. Wear ankle weights.
3. Hold the board in a way that allows you to stand up as straight as possible.
4. Slowly raise both heels off the ground as high as you can comfortably raise them.
5. Then slowly allow your heels to return down.

6. Bring your heals up and down slowly as many times as you can. Start with 20 raises but set a goal to try to do more each week.
7. Breath in and out with each raise to stretch your lungs and add as much oxygen as possible to your body.

Earlier in section 10 (Decompress) I advised that you could go to the deep end of your pool, with your weight on and just hand on your float board without your feet touching the bottom. The weights will stretch your vertebrae's. Well, a great idea is to end your daily program with a decompression stretch. And, as you hang there, let your mind also relax.

CALF RAISES

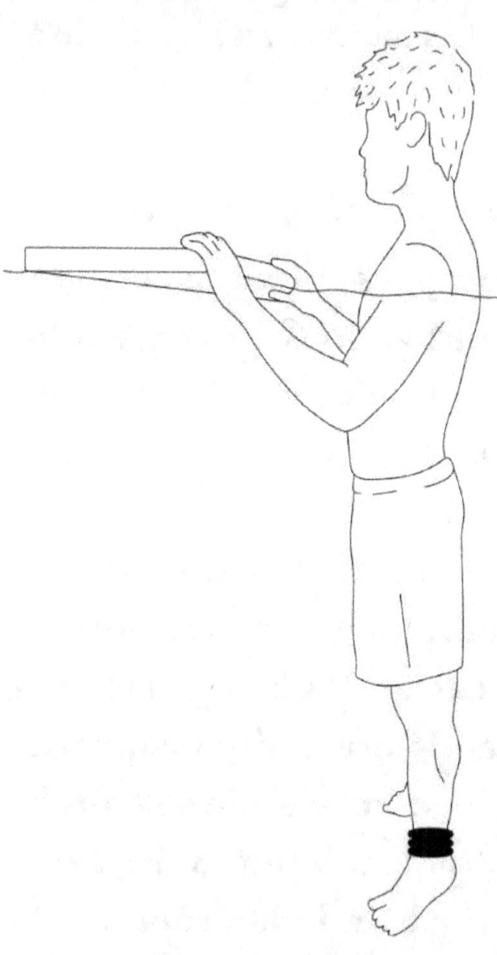

13. Biceps Exercise

This exercise helps build biceps, and it also helps strengthen your core.

Actions:

1. Stand in neck-high or shoulder-high water.

2. Wear ankle weights for greater stability.

3. Bend your knees just a bit to take any stress off your spine.

4. Bring both your arms down to your sides.

5.Cup your hands for resistance.

6.Then extend your arms back as far as they will go, keeping them as straight as you can.

5. Now bring your arms up in a "curling motion" as close to your body until your hands come out of the water. Try to imagine you have a barbell in your hands and are doing conventional arm curls with weights. It's the same motion, but now you'll be doing arm curls in the water, weightless, using water resistance to build your biceps.

6. The reverse of this exercise will help build your forearms and triceps. Start with your cupped hands at the top of the water and then drive your arms down by your sides hard.

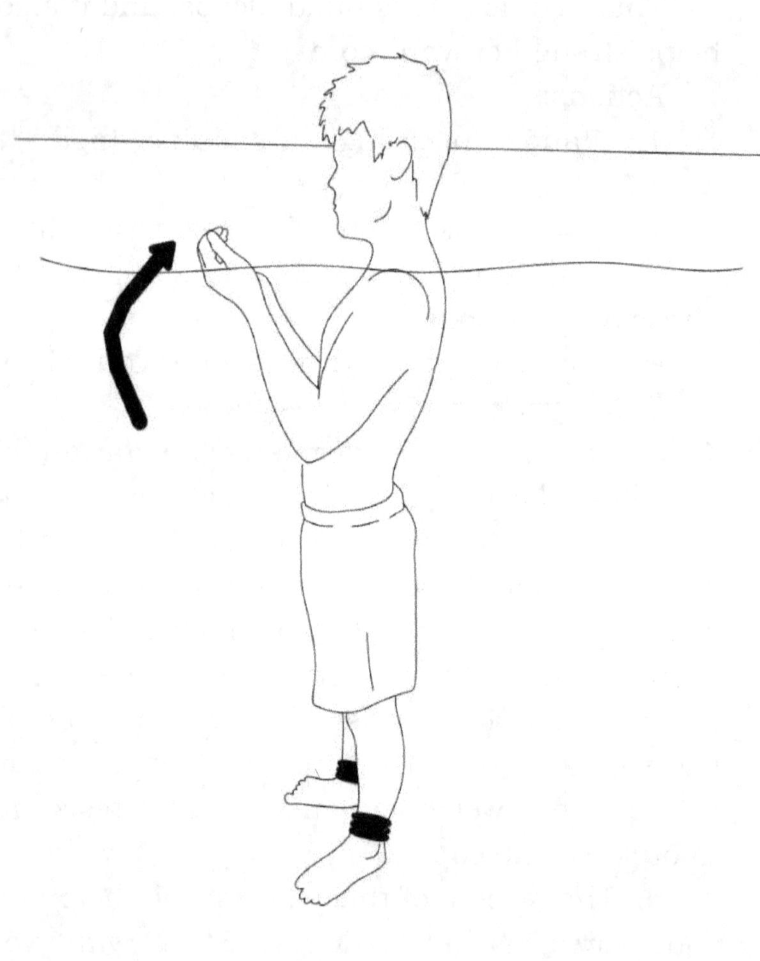

14. Kegel and Stomach Exercise

This exercise will strengthen your pelvic floor and at the same time add strength to your abdominal muscles.

Why would you want to strengthen your pelvic floor if your goal is to primarily strengthen your core? Because doing Kegel exercises and at the same time exercising your stomach muscles is a part of overall core strengthening.

The abdominals are the biggest "helper" muscles to the pelvic floor. They work together to provide support and stability during daily activities (breathing, coughing, movements of the upper and lower body), and sphincteric.

In the case, of older folks or guys who have had prostate cancer and surgery called a prostatectomy, you might experience "leaking" which is called urinary incontinence. But Kegel exercises and the ability to strengthen the pelvic floor significantly helps.

And, if you are a woman who has given birth, it's possible that you too might have leaking issues. Kegel exercises are proven to reduce such a condition.

Other Health Benefits
WEIGHT LOSS

If one of your goals using aqua therapy is to improve your physical health, then consider how you might add to this therapy by weight management if you are overweight. I lost 18 pounds over two years just by increasing my metabolic burn via exercise.

I've been told by many experts that being overweight is a major cause of many physical and health problems. It certainly was not great for my back to carry 50 to 60 pounds of fat around with me that I gained when I stop exercising, So, given my terrible back condition, I was driven to lose weight and as I wrote this book, using only my aqua therapy program, I would like to lose another 20 pounds and am doing that with a combination of diet and exercise.

The average adult burns about 2,000 calories a day doing absolutely nothing. However, if you consume more than 2,000 calories a day, it's more likely than not that you'll gain weight. Sure, increasing your metabolic burn with aqua therapy or other cardiovascular activities that do not stress your bad back will be helpful, but with a bad back.

you'll need to go on a diet with fewer calories to supplement a program using Aqua Therapy to avoid surgery.

People say a big breakfast is the most important meal of the day, but I have totally stopped eating large breakfasts. I do have a cup of coffee, mostly out of habit, but each morning I make a "smoothie" in my Vitamix. Below is the recipe that I use.

John's Healthy Smoothie for Two

1 cup of oat milk
2 scoops Biochem whey protein powder
1 cup Fage 5% Greek Yogurt
1 frozen banana
¾ cup frozen blueberries
¾ cup frozen strawberries
¾ cup frozen cut pineapple
3/4 cup frozen dark pitted cherries
2 pitted dates
2 tablespoons local honey
1 tablespoon coconut oil
2 cups organic baby spinach

I found that this drink gives me more energy than I was getting from a large breakfast that might contain hundreds of calories, and I believe my smoothie has strongly contributed to my weight loss. I have cut lunch (the smoothie normally controls my appetite until dinner), and I have also significantly reduced the portion sizes of my dinners. If my wife and I go out to dinner, we normally order one appetizer and one entree and split them.

Eating smaller portions allows your stomach to shrink a bit, but in time, you really will not feel hungry following dinner. The real test is a desire for snacks during the day, and I found that eating snap peas, carrots, celery, or other raw vegetables can fend off hunger during the day. Another help is to drink a large glass of water when you feel hungry. Water not only fills your stomach, it helps flush your system and remove dead cells and toxins that you might have ingested from the foods you have eaten.

With respect to a total body health program, know that toxins and trace toxins can be found in every food sold today (meat, chicken, vegetables, etc.). All contain trace toxins. Even organic foods contain trace toxins. The only foods you can purchase today that are mostly pure are biodynamic foods.

I didn't know what biodynamic foods were until I did research. I found that it takes about two years for an organic farmer to reconstitute the soil to get all the toxins, and most of the trace toxins ... and even trace metals ... out of the soil.

Then the biodynamic association tests the soil and, if pure, certifies that farmers can claim they grow biodynamic foods.

Google "What are biodynamic foods?" ... and "Why are biodynamic foods better?"

If you do Google biodynamic foods, look for a recent article published in *Shape* magazine. It's quite informative, but one of the statements made was: "Biodynamic farming is a way of viewing a farm as a living organism, self-contained, self-sustaining, and following the cycles of nature," says Elizabeth Candelario, managing director at Demeter, the world's only certifier of biodynamic farms and products. "Think of it as organic—but better."

To find out more, visit White Leaf Provisions ... www.whiteleafprovisions.com; They're doing a great job providing some of the purest foods in America. They specialize in baby foods, but a huge part of their business are vegans and other health minded people who want ultra-healthy snacks for work, hiking, boating, or after a workout.

PREVENT ATROPHY

I personally believe that this section of the book is one of the most important chapters. Why? Because you or someone you know may at some time in your life experience atrophy.

Atrophy is the partial or complete wasting away of a part of the body due to many causes, but the lack of exercise is a major cause.

If you have been confined to a wheelchair, or been in an accident, and have broken a leg, arm, shoulder, hip, or had a surgical operation that resulted in a partial or complete incapacitation over a long period of time during your recovery, you risk having atrophy somewhere in your body.

Your condition might be so severe that you wouldn't consider going to a gym, your yoga class, your physical therapist, or even your chiropractor, but if you have access to either a private or public pool, you might consider aqua therapy ... but only after you obtain clearance from your doctor.

Unless you have an open wound or your doctor has given you specific instructions not to shower, take a bath, or enter a pool, consider aqua therapy during your recovery.

In a pool you're weightless and being weightless significantly reduces the stress on your back, legs, and other parts of your body. Water provides resistance to your arms and legs as you move. But you can control the force of the exercise by simply reducing or increasing the movement of a body part through the water.

Start with a program that allows you to slowly move specific body parts through the water and over time gradually increase that force and the number of repetitions.

Use or modify the exercises found in this book. Under the advice of your physician, create an aqua therapy program what will allow you to strengthen just about every part of your body without causing injury anywhere. You and your doctor can design a specific range of exercises that you can do in a pool to minimize atrophy and hasten your recovery.

BONUS: Aqua Yoga and Aqua Stretching

Aqua yoga and aqua stretching join the mind and body in many ways because they *incorporate* similar movements. Both aqua yoga and aqua stretching involve focusing on proper breathing and allowing your mind to feel the response to each movement. These movements may be accomplished by anyone in a water environment.

Much of what follows in this section has already been described in the aqua therapy section using a float board and ankle weights. Aqua yoga and aqua stretching don't always require a float board or ankle weights; sometimes you may simply hold on to the side of the pool.

Breathing

In aqua yoga and aqua stretching, proper breathing is essential if you wish to achieve the most satisfaction and positive results.

Holding your breath while exercising creates resistance and restricts the amount of oxygen reaching critical parts of your body that are needed to build and strengthen muscles, tendons, and ligaments. So, be sure to breathe properly with each exercise.

I recommend counting. Counting keeps your mind sharp and allows you to perform each exercise to a completed state. It also helps you advance your workouts: "Yesterday I did 10 repetitions and today I'll do 12." Remember, your aqua yoga and aqua stretching exercises can be quite simple and if you keep your daily routine simple, it's much more likely that you will remain injury free.

The Mountain Pose to Perfect Your Breathing

Stand in mid-chest-deep water with your ankle weights on. Form a comfortable stance and bring awareness to your breathing.

Start by breathing in through your nose as deep as you can all the way to your belly. Then slowly allow your breath to exhale through your mouth from your belly. Feel your breath move upward through your chest and finally to your neck, collarbone, and throat. Remember: inhale through your nose and exhale through your mouth. This is as much a "mental exercise" as it is physical. The key to proper breathing while doing aqua yoga, aqua stretching and even aqua therapy is to fill your lungs as far down as possible. Try to imagine that you are bringing air down to your belly. The lower you can bring air into your lungs, the better. Deepwater divers practice deep breathing to expand their lungs before they make their dive. If you wish to test the power of deep breathing, stand in waist high water with your ankle weights on and then go under water without first practicing deep breathing.

While under water, count to yourself. An average person who has not trained in underwater swimming will stay under water for perhaps 15 or 20 seconds. Then come up and practice deep breathing. Breathe in as far as you can and slowly exhale. Do this perhaps five or six times. Then go back under water and count again.

Most people will double their time under water after deep breathing a few times. This exercise stretches your lungs and adds more oxygen to your blood, allowing you to relax more during your workouts.

I enjoy counting as I breathe in and breathe out. Try it first with a count of three as you breathe in and a count of three as you breathe out. This creates a pace that's even. And as you get better, you can increase your pace with a count of four in and four out. Deepwater divers have counts above 10 in and 10 out because they have developed their lungs over time.

My friend, John Doolittle, who is a Navy Seal and mentioned in the acknowledgement section of this book, can stay underwater for over three minutes. When I started my program, I could only hold my breath for about a minute. But as I write this book I broke my record and stayed under water for three minutes ... but realize I have been practicing beating Doolittle for over two years.

Breath practice will also calm the mind and prepare your body for deeper stretches. In the Mountain Pose, as you breathe in through your nose, try to mentally lengthen your spine by standing taller.

Then bring your shoulders down and away from your ears as you breathe out through your mouth.

However, focus on how other areas of your body are feeling as you start to enter a mind-body connection.

Still in your Mountain Pose, inhale again through your nose and extend your arms and palms from beside your body straight up and overhead. Then exhale through your mouth and reverse your arms back down slowly to your sides. As you are doing this movement, you may combine it with very slow head turns and shoulder rolls that will help relax your head, but strengthen your neck, and shoulders.

It's well known throughout the health and fitness world that exercise is one of the most important—perhaps *the* most important—things we can do to maintain good health.

In the case of aqua yoga and aqua stretching, these exercises will not only keep you fit for your daily life, but after illness or even surgery, they can dramatically increase the speed of your recovery.

As an example, a surgeon can operate to repair part of your body, and nature will heal you after surgery, but during that process, your body will start to atrophy, and you can lose muscle tone and ligament flexibility. On land, it will be difficult to regain your muscle tone and ligament flexibility while you are recuperating, but in the water, your recovery will be far easier and safer.

Upper Back Stretch/Leg Stretch

For a shoulder stretch, raise your arms up into a goal-post position with elbows bent to 90 degrees. Then you're your arms back on each side. You should feel a pull across your upper back.

Another option is to interlace the fingers behind the head. Then pull your elbows back. You should feel a pull across your chest.

For a leg stretch, bring one leg back behind you, but keep it straight. Then push forward and bend the front knee of that leg. Keep your back leg straight as you bend the front knee forward 90 degrees.

Balance

Balance is of critical importance in both land and pool exercise. However, the pool is a great place to practice balance because you'll feel safer and grow more confidence in your balancing skills. Falls during exercise or sports attribute to many injuries which we all want to avoid. However, in a pool, it's far less likely that you will sustain a fall injury. Balance can be developed in a pool by simply standing on one foot and raising the other off the bottom of the pool.

Start by using a pool noodle, or a float board ... or simply by making small figure eights (sculling) with your hands in the water to help stabilize you.

If you're in a Mountain Pose, try to lift one foot and not fall over. Try first with one foot and then the other.

Of interest, many people can balance better with one foot than the other. However, with practice, you'll get better with both feet.

Yoga Tree Pose

Standing in a Mountain Pose with sculling hands out to your sides to maintain balance, bring the sole of one foot to the inside of the calf or thigh of the other. Then allow your bent knee to open to the outside of your body. Be sure to breathe as identified above, because holding your breath will make balancing harder. This is a great hip and inner thigh stretch too.

As your balance improves, you may bring one hand out of the water like a branch of a tree while still maintaining your foot position on the inside of your other calf or thigh. For more intensity you may bring both hands out of the water toward the sky.

Practice this as it will take time to become proficient. Continue to breathe, keeping a standing tall alignment.

You may practice this with or without ankle weights; try it and see which fits your needs better.

Remember, aqua yoga and aqua stretching can become your link between a sedentary lifestyle and a healthier, active life. These exercises allow you to transition from a relaxed state to one where you can advance to more active activities, such as bike riding, yard work, tennis, running, and so many other things without unnecessary strain and without the risk of injury. The prevention of simple sports injuries such as knee pain, shoulder pain, and even tennis elbow can be increased in many cases by regular yoga and stretching, regardless of whether you are using a pool or not.

Shoulder Stretch/Half Dog

Place both hands on the side of the pool in shallow water, walk your feet back away from your hands on the wall by hinging at your hips toward a 90-degree position, but keeping your legs and back straight. Allow your hips to move back feeling a stretch in the shoulders, hips, back and hamstrings.

You may like to move your head as if looking under your arm towards your neck to feel a nice neck stretch and observe which side of your neck feels tighter. That's the side to work on more. It's important that you know that with both aqua yoga and aqua stretching you should not try to achieve any movement to a maximum level. Over-stretching is dangerous and totally unnecessary.

The trick is to perform each exercise in a peaceful and relaxing way. Start slowly and let your body gain the benefits over time, but if you wish to improve quickly, then perform your exercises on a more regular basis. It's important to listen to your body as it will tell you your limits. Never push beyond the point where your body tells you it hurts. Most importantly, I think you will be amazed after you create your own plan for both aqua yoga and aqua stretching and notice that after each session you'll feel more relaxed, and your mind will seem sharper.

Side Stretch/Yoga Triangle

In the shallow part of your pool, take a wide stance, adjust your left foot to point to the side of your body, keeping both legs straight. Then reach your left arm down toward the pool bottom and lift the other arm toward the sky. Allow your hips to move slightly toward the back leg, feeling the great stretch along the back side of your body. You may bend the back elbow and place your hand beside your ear to take any stress off that shoulder. Repeat the movement on the other side and observe how it may feel different.

Standing Calf Stretch

Be sure both your feet are pointing forward and not to one side or the other. Then facing and leaning forward, hold on to the side of the pool, move one leg back until it's straight. Bring the other leg forward and bend that knee slightly.

Slowly move your hips forward, keeping you back leg straight. Do not lift that back foot. As your hips move forward, you should feel a stretch in your calf muscle. Hold that stretch for about three breaths. Do not over-stretch. Then switch legs.

Heel Raise/Elevated Mountain

This is identified above using the float board and ankle weights, but it can also be done holding on to the side of the pool. With both feet facing forward, simply raise up towards your toes so that your heels leave the pool floor. Move slowly up and slowly down. Start with only 10 repetitions, but, over time, advance to as many as you feel comfortable. This not only builds your calf muscles but increases the flexibility in your ankles all the way to your toes.

Low Back Stretch/Camel Pose

Standing upright with knees slightly bent to take pressure off your back, bring both arms around the sides of your waist in the area of your lower back. Place your hands against your lower back and gently push forward while pulling both shoulders back. This will allow your hips to move forward while slightly arching your back. You should feel your shoulders also moving slightly down and back. Keep your neck relaxed looking forward or slightly upward. If you are prone to back pain, especially after sitting in a work chair for a long period, this is a wonderful exercise to help you maintain better back function.

Final Relaxation Pose

Now is time to let go and use your breathing to evoke a deep relaxation response.

Without your ankle weights, find a comfortable relaxing position. Pool noodles may be placed under your arms and wrap around behind your back. Use as many as you like to support and float your upper body.

Resting back into the noodle, allow your legs and arms to relax as you float. Close your eyes if that is comfortable. Breathe in slowly, relax your energy, and exhale away any tension or cares that may be on your mind.

Allow yourself 10 minutes or more to just be peaceful and relaxed in the pool.

Conclusion

As I conclude this book, it's hard to believe I'm the same man I was just two years ago, when I couldn't even walk to the mailbox and back. Back then I was facing my third back surgery ... one could have left me a cripple in a wheelchair. Today, there's a spring in my step. Now, I'm back to doing many of the activities I love, like working in the yard and enjoying long walks. I may never be a champion athlete again, but now I am nearly pain free, thanks to aqua therapy and the exercises I've outlined in this book.

Your first step is to take this book to your physician. Let your physician look at these exercises and give you advice about whether aqua therapy is right for you. Then and only then should you attempt the exercises in this book.

But I hope you can and that you *will.* Preventing surgery is huge. Getting in better shape has so many wonderful benefits! Losing weight, being healthier...this is what happened to me after developing my program. I believe you'll benefit as well.

Of course, I can't *guarantee* these exercises will work for you, but I can guarantee one thing: If you try these exercises for six months, you might not get better, but you *will* get a lot *cleaner!*

Best of luck, *John M. Capozzi*

About the Author

John M. Capozzi served in the military during the Vietnam war. Following his discharge from the military, he began his career with American Airlines in operations and was promoted eight times in eight years, leaving as a Director of Marketing in its corporate headquarters.

He then joined a division of the Midland Bank Group as vice president of sales for its North American operating company. He was promoted five times in five years, leaving as the North American CEO. He served on the company board and the board of its Travelers Cheque division.

John was one of the organizers of The Presidents' Summit for America's Future, which was Chaired by President George H. W. Bush (41) and by Secretary of State Colin Powell. This effort became America's Promise. An Alliance, dedicated to assisting high-risk children. John has been mentoring inner city children for more than 30 years.

During this period, he worked with the Points of Light Foundation, which was chaired by President George H. W. Bush.

Additionally, John was one of the creators and funding sources for the Smoke Free Society Campaign with the U.S. Surgeon General, Dr. C. Everett Koop. John's mother and father both died from lung disease. They were lifelong smokers.

That campaign resulted in the government putting labels on cigarette packs that say, "Cigarettes can cause lung cancer." He tried to get the FDS to ban cigarettes, but the tobacco growing lobby was too strong even though hundreds of thousands of people have died from lung cancer. He went on The Today Show to promote that campaign with Charlotte Ford ... Henry Ford's daughter who served on his board.

He then funded and formed Shape Up America with the U.S. Surgeon General and launched this national initiative at the White House with Hillary Clinton. Then obesity in America was at 30%. As this book is written it's now at 70%.

He is an accomplished entrepreneur, having successfully started and sold over 20 companies in his career. One was a "healthy" food company that he built to over $50 million in three years and sold to one of the largest food companies in America.

John served for nine years on the Business School Board of Fairfield University, for two years on the board of the Enterprise Center at Yale University, and on the board of Greens Farms Academy in Westport, CT, for six years. He also served on the Board of Operation Independence for the State of Israel for 14 years. He has been a speaker at many events and colleges and has appeared on the Today Show and on Good Morning America. He was the youngest Eagle Scout in New York State history.

John has been a professional skier, a tournament squash and tennis player, a marathon runner, and an avid golfer.

He is also the author of seven books. There are over 15 million copies of his hard cover and mini books in circulation.

Acknowledgments

To create this book and to verify that my aqua therapy program is accurate, I sought opinions from several health care professionals who I highly respect for their medical training, yoga skills, physical therapy, and fitness knowledge.

In two cases, these exceptional advisors also incurred their own major personal injuries, and their recovery experiences were invaluable to my ability to avoid major surgery. I cannot thank the following advisors enough for saving the quality of my life.

DR. BRAD LERNER.

Dr. Lerner is my family's primary physician. He built a wonderful concierge practice, **Lerner Cohen Concierge Healthcare**, located in Sarasota, Florida. I have taken the time to identify Dr. Lerner in detail in this book, because to have a doctor of his quality endorse this work is beyond amazing, and I hope gives the reader comfort that the content of my book is sound.

His firm is a private, primary care practice that maintains time-tested relationships with trusted specialists who meet his firm's exacting standards of knowledge, service, and compassion. When my wife and I moved from Connecticut ten years ago we selected Dr. Lerner after an extensive review of many physicians in Florida and doing so has proved to be one of the best decisions we have ever made.

No matter what our medical issues are (dental, eye care, dental, dermatology, etc.), Dr. Lerner has researched, vetted, and introduced us to "the very best doctors" in our area, and, in some cases, in other parts of Florida.

Doctor Lerner completed his undergraduate studies at Johns Hopkins University with a B.A. degree in Biological Chemistry in 1975, where he was elected to the Phi Beta Kappa Honor Society. He then attended the University of Florida College of Medicine, where he was elected to the Alpha Omega Alpha Honor Medical Society and received his M.D. degree in 1979.

He then completed his Internal Medicine internship and residency at The University of North Carolina at Chapel Hill, North Carolina Dr. Lerner relocated to Sarasota in 1982 to join Drs. William Deports, Burt Veazey, and Duncan Finlay in their well-respected medical practice.

He became certified by the American Board of Internal Medicine in 1982.

He served as Chief of Internal Medicine at Sarasota Memorial Hospital and was a member of its Medical Executive Committee for many years. He is widely respected by his peers in the Sarasota community as both an outstanding clinician and a leader in the local healthcare market.

In 1994 Dr. Lerner was responsible for the creation of Sarasota Memorial Hospital's only primary care group, later to be named First Physicians Group.

He served as Chief Medical Administrative Officer (CMAO) of First Physicians Group from its inception in 1994 until 2005. In this role, He led a group of close to 50 physicians and 250 employees, while maintaining his Internal Medicine practice and working closely with the administration and board of Sarasota Memorial Hospital. He left First Physicians Group in 2005 to partner with his long- time friend and colleague Dr. Louis Cohen in the creation of Lerner Cohen Concierge Healthcare.

Professionally, he can devote his full attention to the distinct needs of his patients with a strong emphasis on wellness and prevention ... all while providing an unsurpassed level of access and care.

While I wish to thank him for his exceptional advice with respect to my back issues, I also wish to thank him for his professional care of my wife, who suffers from devastating long term side effects from Covid 19. I believe Dr. Lerner saved her life during a most difficult time in our 56-year marriage.

AUSTIN JENSEN

Austin (CSCA, PTA, LMT) has helped me recover from past surgeries. He was a Division I football player who was in a near-fatal auto accident. He fractured his skull in two places, suffering two subdural hematomas (brain bleeds), fractured his pelvis in four places, and was put in a medically induced coma in intensive care for weeks. His hip and leg muscles suffered damage and he had significant pain in his lower back in combination with post-concussion syndrome and vertigo.

A month after his accident, Austin began extensive physical therapy, and was introduced to "muscular re-education" to strengthen his core and re-build his body.

In about six months of almost daily therapy, Austin had rebuilt the muscles in his core and was back to his normal physical condition and full training regime to get back on the football field ... only to be declined the opportunity to play again due to his traumatic brain injuries that he suffered in his auto accident.

Two years later, in 2012, Austin began assisting patients as a strength coach and licensed massage therapist (LMT).

He was certified by The National Strength and Conditioning Association, a certification that requires a bachelor's degree in Exercise Science and Health Promotion.

Initially Austin started working with athletes and special population patients/clients (post-rehab, stroke, Parkinson's, and acute and chronic rehab patients). In 2015, Austin obtained his license in physical therapy (PTA).

He utilizes a unique approach to each of his clients, curating from his background as a Division I athlete, strength and conditioning specialist, massage therapist, and former critical care patient to help others achieve wellness and become the best version of themselves.

Austin's position as a former critical care patient allows him to put himself in the shoes of his current clients/patients, working from a compassionate, comprehensive, and motivational aspect of healthcare and athletics. His website is ABetterYouPerformance.com.

JEA COFFMAN.

For the past nine years, my wife has used the personal training services of Jea Coffman, who comes to our home twice a week. Jea is dedicated to teaching and training clients in Southwest Florida, in fitness support, wellness, and rehabilitation from injury. Jea had a significant career with the United States Army in fitness and wellness, including serving in Iraq and assisting disabled veterans,. She is a Certified Personal Trainer and a ERYT Yoga Instructor. Her website is ThaiYogaFit.com.

CAPTAIN JOHN DOOLITTLE.

John is a personal friend and fellow "warrior." He started his military career at the United States Air Force Academy and achieved the rank of Captain.

However, he wanted to do more for his country, so in 1992 he left the Air Force to join the Navy to become a Navy SEAL. He then again achieved the rank of Captain and served with SEAL Team TWO as a Navy Seal.

Before the 9/11 terrorist attack on our World Trade Center, he commanded the security team for President George W. Bush during his trip to Kosovo.

John deployed to Afghanistan, Iraq, and several other hot spots around the world with our Navy SEALs following 9/11.

One of the most amazing things about Captain Doolittle is that after he lost a fellow SEAL in combat, he decided to swim across the English Channel to honor the memory of his teammate and raise money for the Navy SEAL Foundation. The temperature was below 60 degrees, and he only wore a Speedo.

He commented: "I was in terrific pain and was about to give up, but when I looked over at the chase boat and I saw my dad and my support team holding the American flag, and I knew that I had to finish." That's the mark of a true patriot.

Following an injury during his military service, John discovered and used KAATSU for his incredible recovery from a broken back. K A A T S U was invented in Japan but engineered and designed in California.

This incredible technology is the pioneer in the emerging Blood Flow Restriction (BFR) market that automatically and safely optimizes blood circulation for health, fitness, rehabilitation, and recovery.

KAATSU utilizes small, automated compressor and pneumatic stretchable bands, which are placed around your arms or legs.

The bands inflate and deflate in a patented sequence based on algorithms that boost circulation, improve hormonal balance, and develop muscle tone in a time-effective manner with a minimum of effort. KAATSU equipment and proprietary protocols offer unparalleled performance, precision, and safety for users of all ages, fitness levels, and walks of life. It can be used anywhere anytime to help you recover faster, rehab stronger and perform better. John is a senior officer in this company.

KAATSU is used by many major professional sports teams, as well as members of the U.S. Olympic Team for performance enhancement.

You can read more about KAATSU at www.kaatsu.com.

DR. BRUCE BECKER.

I cannot thank Dr. Becker enough for his advice and for providing the Foreword to my book.

Following graduation from Tulane University School of Medicine, Dr. Becker completed his residency training in Physical Medicine and Rehabilitation at the University of Washington.

He was an Associate Professor at Wayne State University School of Medicine and served as Vice President of Medical Affairs for the Rehabilitation Institute of Michigan from January 1992 until June of 1998, when he moved to Spokane to serve as the Medical Director of St. Luke's Rehabilitation Institute. He served at St. Luke's until January of 2006.

Dr. Becker holds clinical appointments as a Clinical Professor in the Department of Rehabilitation Medicine at the University of Washington School of Medicine and was previously Research Professor at Washington State University where he founded and was the Director of the National Aquatic & Sports Medicine Institute. This is where he pursued physiological research during aquatic activity. In January of 2012, he was appointed the Director of Health Benefit Research Programs for the National Swimming Pool Foundation.

However, in 1997, Dr. Andrew Cole and Dr. Becker co-authored the textbook *Comprehensive Aquatic Therapy,* which was published by Butterworth-Heinemann. *Comprehensive Aquatic Therapy* was published in Portuguese and German.

Elsevier then published the second edition of the textbook in 2002. A third edition was published in 2011 by Washington State

University Press in English and Chinese. There are other translations in progress.

Of importance, Dr. Becker has published numerous chapters on aquatic therapy in most of the leading textbooks in rehabilitation medicine. Further, he has authored aquatic research articles in major medical journals and has lectured globally on aquatic health benefits and rehabilitation.

He has been honored by several organizations for pioneering the value of aquatic activity and exercise. In 1999, he Aquatic Therapy and Rehabilitation Institute named Dr. Becker as the Aquatic Professional of the year.

Aquatics International magazine named Dr. Becker to the Power 25 in 2006 and again in 2011. He was the recipient of the John K. Williams, Jr. International Adapted Aquatics Award from the International Swimming Hall of Fame in May of 2011 for his work in adapted aquatics.

Dr. Becker has been the recipient of aquatic research grants from the National Swimming Pool Foundation, as well as the recipient of other grants from The National Institute of Disability and Rehabilitation Research of the Department of Education.

KELLIE FOX.

Kellie has been a Physical Therapist since 1991. She earned her associate degree in medical assisting from Erie Community College in Williamsville, NY, and a bachelor's degree in science/PT in Troy, NY.

She has experience working in various health related settings, including inpatients, outpatients, rehab, home care, hospice, and long-term care. Over the past 20 years, Kellie has specialized in Pelvic Floor Rehabilitation with training from Herman & Wallace Pelvic Rehabilitation Institute and The American Physical Therapy Association.

In her free time, Kellie volunteers for nonprofit organizations assisting those in need.

She is an accomplished athlete and participates in biking, swimming, jogging, dancing, yoga, weight training, and pickleball. Kellie has been invaluable in her help as an expert in urinary incontinence improvement and core strengthening.